The Pliocene Diet

A Guide to Healthy Ancestral Eating

By

ALICE DEE

ALICE DEE

First Edition

Copyright © 2023 Alice Dee

Published by Raw From the Garden Press

Visit these websites for related books and information:

www.PlioceneDiet.com

www.NutritionalHealer.com

www.TheFoodForestGuide.com

www.PeakPerformanceDiet.com

www.RawFromTheGarden.com

www.RawVeganRecipesBook.com

ISBN: 9798873185672

DEDICATION

This book is dedicated to the love of my life and my beloved pack. I feel honored to live and run with you.

ACKNOWLEDGEMENTS

I want to thank and acknowledge the contributions to this book made by Poffo Ortiz and Grimarthar Ceikeverjn. I also want to thank my dear family and the love of my life for supporting and encouraging me throughout the process of researching and writing this book.

TABLE OF CONTENTS

PREFACE

Welcome to "The Pliocene Diet: A Guide to Healthy Ancestral Eating", a detailed and science-based exploration into the rejuvenating world of ancestral nutrition. In an era inundated with fad dietary trends and conflicting nutritional advice, this book aims to guide you back to the scientific roots of our evolutionary past—the Pliocene epoch.

As we embark on this dietary study together, you will first be introduced to the fundamental principles of the Pliocene Diet, drawing on the intuitive food-wisdom of our ancient hominid ancestors and our closest wild-living great ape relatives to inform our modern approach to nutrition. In doing so, this book serves not just as a diet guide, but also as a captivating narrative that intertwines the science of nutrition with human evolutionary history and practical dietary wisdom to invite readers to reconnect with the inherent knowledge imprinted in our genetic heritage.

After laying the groundwork for this exploration and setting the stage for the enlightening chapters that follow, Chapter 2's entry into the science of nutrition delves into the scientific underpinnings of the Pliocene Diet, bridging the gap between contemporary nutritional understanding and the dietary wisdom of our ancestors.

Chapter 3 then compares ancestral to modern diets, offering a compelling juxtaposition of the dietary landscapes of yesteryears and today, providing a context for the necessity of revisiting our nutritional roots. The ensuing Chapters 4 and 5 on dietary principles and food choices suitable for the Pliocene Diet delve into the core ideas and specific food recommendations to help demystify the essence of healthy ancestral eating.

In Chapter 6, this book addresses additional facets of the Pliocene Diet, with the goal of widening your perspective on creating holistic well-being.

Chapter 7 then brings practicality into play, offering insights into preparing nourishing meals aligned with our ancestral heritage, while Chapter 8, acts as a guide for those embarking on this transformative dietary journey to better health. Following this, you then get tangible support with meal plans and recipes in Chapters 9 and 10 to help ensure that your transition to the Pliocene Diet is not only healthful but also inspiring, delicious and sustainable.

As you immerse yourself in the pages that follow, let this book be your compass in navigating the realm of ancestral nutrition. May it empower you to make better-informed choices and reconnect with the ancient food wisdom encoded in our very DNA as you embark on a dietary path toward vibrant health, well-being and longevity.

To your health!

Alice Dee

THE PLIOCENE DIET

CHAPTER 1: INTRODUCTION

As you will learn from this book, the human digestive physiology and circulatory system that evolved during the Pliocene Epoch that stretched from 5.3 to 2.6 million years ago is best suited for eating raw whole plant foods our hominid ancestors foraged in the wild.

Not only does this most natural ancestral diet for humans not include any significant amount of animal products, it even excludes consuming more modern agriculturally-grown plants seeds like grains and legumes that can cause some people to suffer digestive issues.

Modern Human Diets Compared to the Pliocene and Great Ape Diet

Despite widespread human omnivorous behavior in the modern era, our actual human physiology has never adapted to allow us to thrive while consuming the meat that can only be provided by relatively modern technologies. Humans need unnatural things like weapons to hunt animals or kill them in slaughterhouses, tools to cut chunks of flesh from dead animal bodies, fire to cook animal flesh to make it edible, and herbs and/or plant-derived condiments to make it palatable, but all of this relatively modern technology still does not make consuming meat healthy for us. Most of us would even feel disgusted at the very thought of eating raw unseasoned flesh torn from an animal's body with our teeth, a sentiment that no truly carnivorous or omnivorous animal likely experiences.

While certain algaes and seaweeds make nutritious food for humans that we can easily obtain from oceans, lakes and waterways and consume in their natural raw state, humans are clearly not adapted to catch or consume fish or shellfish and prepare the flesh of such creatures for safe consumption. To do so, humans require unnatural tools like fishing rods, hooks, nets, knives, traps, and cooking implements. Also, instead of eating the flesh and bones of fish raw, which most will find unappetizing, humans usually remove bones and then cook and season the flesh with plant foods we actually do find appetizing like herbs, lemon and ginger. Fish and shellfish therefore cannot be included among the foods humans are naturally adapted to consume.

Also, our mammalian Pliocene era ancestors certainly drank breast milk from their mothers in infancy before the age of weaning, as many human babies do today. That completely natural behavior remains a far cry from consuming significant amounts of saturated fat-laden dairy products coming from disease-ridden factory farms well into adulthood. Furthermore, the tragic elements of dairy food production include the inhumane and traumatic stealing of babies from their mothers, as well as the tight confinement and cruel killing of almost all male babies since they do not give milk. Even the females abused in dairy production are slaughtered at a fraction of their natural lifespan once their milk production slows sufficiently to make feeding and housing them uneconomic for the profit-hungry factory farmer.

The dairy industry only uses female cows, known as heifers, for milk production. A cow only produces milk during the first year of its calf's life, with an ideal lactation period of 10 months. However, in many instances, this period extends beyond 10 months, followed by a two-month dry period before the next calving. To maintain a consistent milk supply, dairy farmers often use artificial insemination which is the ethical equivalent of rape since the cows do not participate voluntarily in this sexually-invasive process that results in a burdensome forced pregnancy.

Cows trapped in the dairy industry typically have an average lifespan of only around six years, which is a small fraction of the 20 to 25 years they could ordinarily live. After this short period during which they undergo repeated rape, forced pregnancy, excessive milking from oversized mammary glands, and the traumatic theft and killing of their babies, they are generally slaughtered themselves for low-quality meat if they do not die earlier from abuse, disease or neglect. The typical age of death in the dairy industry ranges from four to seven years old.

When it comes to eggs, some wild-living great apes may consume the occasional wild bird egg, although this generally makes up a trivial and non-essential part of their diet, and our Pliocene era ancestors may have done the same. Still, that rare behavior does not compare in magnitude to the number of eggs that many humans regularly consume today, each of which contains a huge amount of artery-clogging cholesterol and saturated fat. Also, the nutritional content of an occasional wild-laid bird egg would have been notably better than that which can currently be derived from the poor quality eggs over-produced by chickens cruelly caged in battery factory farms today.

From an ethical standpoint, egg production is fraught with cruel and indecent practices. Male chicks, deemed economically worthless, meet a brutal end through grinding, a method where they are systematically crushed alive shortly after hatching. For the egg-laying hens, the lifetime confinement in small battery cages becomes their grim reality. These cramped, barren enclosures deprive them of the most basic behavioral expressions, stifling their natural instincts and well-being. The toll of captivity extends further into the ubiquitous practice of painfully debeaking birds without anesthetic and the unnerving phenomenon of cannibalism, a sad consequence of the stressful and overcrowded conditions these birds are forced to endure.

Even more tragic is the premature cyclical termination of the entire egg-laying flock's existence. At a mere fraction of their natural life span of 10 to 20 years, these fully-sentient beings are routinely killed en masse at less than two years of age. This grim fate is a testament to the egg industry's callous prioritization of profit over compassion, as the lives of these intelligent and sensitive creatures are cut short for mere economic efficiency. The outrageously cruel practices inherent in the egg industry underscore the urgent need for conscientious consideration of the ethical implications of our food choices, challenging us to reevaluate the systems that perpetuate such suffering.

Furthermore, the human digestion and circulatory system have just never evolved sufficiently to make consuming animal foods like meat, dairy and eggs that are very heavy in saturated fat and cholesterol healthy for us. This unnatural behavior tragically results in chronic human diseases like heart disease, strokes, Type II diabetes, cancer, impotence, auto-immune diseases, arthritis and obesity. Also, most people with a conscience do not feel very good about sourcing items from the cruel, disease-ridden and overcrowded animal factory farms and the horrifically violent slaughterhouses that provide those unhealthy animal products to grocery stores in the modern era.

While developing the technology to provide flesh foods to hungry hominids may have initially promoted our ancestors' survival as a species when their forest homes turned into plains as a result of climate change, it unfortunately left us divorced from our most natural and healthiest ancestral diet that evolved during the Pliocene epoch and was based almost exclusively on plant foods. This is the same healthful diet rich in raw plant foods that modern-day great apes like gorillas, bonobos and orangutans still follow in their natural forest environments today.

Humans Can Learn From What Other Great Apes Eat

In contrast to the herbivores that generally eat grass, great apes like humans should ideally base most of their natural diet on fruits. This puts them in a special physiological dietary category known as the frugivores. In addition to fruit, wild-living great apes should and typically do eat a substantial amount of tender green plants; a modest amount of nuts and seeds; small quantities of bark and pith; and a few insects. They sometimes also eat root vegetables, but this is done mainly to prevent starvation when their preferred foods are scarce.

Curiously, great apes might also eat the feces of their own species, which is probably done to populate their gut flora. Feces are also a notable source of the essential vitamin B12 that comes from microbes. The intestinal bacteria commonly hosted by great apes in their hindgut (which includes the lower half of the large intestine or colon) do produce vitamin B12, but it does not get absorbed there. Feces can therefore be re-ingested by great apes to make that essential vitamin available for absorption by the intrinsic factor-mediated mechanism that exclusively occurs in the ileum (the last part of the small intestine).

Great apes can also get the minuscule amount of vitamin B12 they need from eating insects, which they sometimes do in very small amounts when living wild. Modern humans will probably find both of these behaviors unappetizing, so they can instead ingest a vitamin B12 supplement or a multivitamin that contains the 2.4 micrograms of B12 adults need per day to achieve the same goal our wild-living cousins do naturally by consuming feces and bugs.

Great apes also eat small amounts of tree bark, although some people might not be aware that the bark of certain trees, such as pine, spruce, elm, fir, tamarack and birch trees, is indeed edible for humans. Tree bark can actually be a life-saving food when people are starving and have nothing else to eat, as many Scandinavians are aware due to their cultural practice of combining soft pine tree bark with rye flour in times of famine to make bark bread.

Other great apes already understand that tree bark can supply them with some sustenance in a survival situation since the starches and sugars in a tree's bark provide energy for their bodies that can also nourish humans. Since some tree barks are more edible than others, those looking to include tree bark in their diet can look for barks that contain less of the tannins that are highly astringent and can cause constipation, such as cherry and oak bark. If they are looking to slow their digestion down, however, then they can consume herbs higher in tannins like green tea.

Since eating tree bark has some nuances to it that most people today were never taught, it requires some education on how to do it properly and safely. Usually, the most edible part of tree bark for humans is the cambium, which is the tender layer between the xylem or wood and the phloem (inner bark), although the phloem itself is also edible. Humans should therefore focus on eating the nutritious soft inner tree bark instead of the harder outer tree bark that is basically indigestible.

For a refreshing and nutritious snack, the cambium tissue of a tree's bark can be eaten raw, although care needs to be taken to remove it in a way that will not kill the tree, making future harvesting impossible. Eating cambium does involve some exercise for the jaws, and you'll probably want to spit out the stringy parts that remain after the nutritious juices have been sucked out.

Great apes also eat small amounts of pith, which consists of the usually-continuous central strand of spongy tissue found in the stems of most vascular plants that probably serves mainly in nutrient storage. Vascular plants are characterized by the presence of conducting tissue. Examples include the Tracheophyta, such as ferns, horsetails and club mosses, as well as the Spermatophyta, which include conifers, cycads and flowering plants.

This book will show you how to enjoy plant-based nourishment the Pliocene way by consuming the most natural and nutrient-dense foods on the planet. You can literally eat your way to good health by seeking out nature's most nourishing foods for your species.

Natural Nourishment and Lifestyle Elements

The nutrients you put into your body can have a huge effect on your overall well-being. They are also the biggest determinant of how much energy you have throughout the day. Community, movement, sunlight and finding your purpose are also critical lifestyle elements that can enhance your life, although the single greatest factor in human health and disease is how you eat.

Plants offer the most nutrient-dense natural foods humans can eat, and their wide range of phytonutrients was uniquely treasured and sought out by our Pliocene ancestors. You just cannot beat plant-derived foods for the best human nourishment available in the most efficient way when it comes to the least nutrients, water, energy and environmental pollution required to bring them to your table.

If you get one thing right when it comes to your diet, focus on becoming passionate about the quality of the plant foods you gather and eat. This will result in profound positive change in your overall health that will cascade into all of the other areas of your life. When you consume the highest quality, organically grown and non-genetically modified plant foods in their natural raw state, as our Pliocene ancestors did by foraging for them in the wild, you will thrive.

Focus on Consuming the Best Human Nourishment on the Planet

Plants are the absolute center of the ancestral hominid diet that predominated in the Pliocene era. Plants still provide modern humans with the greatest degree of vitality and vigor, and they offer the most efficient and compassionate way of eating for humans.

Some plant foods and/or their components have also been unjustly maligned by the mainstream media based on misleading epidemiology, which is the study of the patterns, causes and effects of health and disease conditions in defined populations. This misinformation is actively promoted by the cruel and polluting animal agriculture industry, and it can cause much harm when people take it as truth if it convinces them to continue to consume animal products in violation of their fundamental nature as frugivores.

As the related sciences of nutritional healing and herbology teach, plants contain a wide spectrum of nutritious and medicinal substances that offer healing qualities for many individuals. Nutritional biochemistry also shows that natural plant-derived whole foods provide the human body with all of the nutrients it needs to thrive. For the best results, you will generally want to look for organically-grown plant foods sourced from your own garden or from the finest organic farms on the planet.

What a beautifully elegant truth it is that everything, every vitamin, mineral, peptide, protein and cofactor that the human body needs to function optimally can be obtained from consuming plants, basking in sunshine and eating the products of microbes you can easily obtain from nutritional yeast and vitamin B12 supplements. Your impressively healthy Pliocene ancestors knew all this instinctively, but it's a key idea that has been lost in recent generations, leading to the profoundly adverse and even deadly health effects seen within modern human cultures that over-eat processed, genetically-modified plant foods and animal products.

Tragically, over 40% of humans living in the United States now meet the formal criteria for obesity, while only an elite 12% of the U.S. population can truly be considered metabolically healthy. (See CDC Obesity Report 2017-2018, Metabolically Unhealthy and its related web page of Adult Obesity Facts[1]) . Like our Pliocene ancestors, modern plant-based dieters employ the sole dietary pattern associated with a normal, healthy body weight as determined by the Body Mass Index or BMI. The BMI is calculated by taking a person's weight in kilograms and dividing that by the square of their height in meters. A high BMI indicates a high degree of body fat that is generally associated with obesity.

It is no exaggeration that this obesity epidemic exists mainly because

---

[1] https://www.cdc.gov/obesity/data/adult.html

humans have forsaken the nutritional wisdom of our Pliocene era ancestors. Humans have traded the foraged plant foods that make us thrive for chronic disease-causing animal foods and ultra-processed carbohydrates, sugars and vegetable oils that invariably lead to smoldering inflammation. This underlies the rampant epidemics of autoimmunity and chronic disease humanity now faces as a greater human tribe.

Correcting Dietary Missteps by Remembering Ancestral Wisdom

Ceasing to consume all animal products is a great start on the way to achieving excellent health, but it's really only part of the nutritional equation. To truly obtain all of the nutrients you need to thrive, organic raw plant foods are a key part of a healthy diet. Processed and cooked foods may provide macronutrients, minerals and calories, but they are often very lacking in the ephemeral micro-nutrients and fiber that promote good health. Also, mass-produced non-organic plant foods may offer less nutrition, while including a slew of potentially harmful chemicals used as pesticides and fertilizers.

In this book, you will find a wealth of information about all the nutrients that are uniquely found in meaningful quantities in plant food and how these special minerals and organic compounds help vitalize us. Although some items that our Pliocene ancestors ate and our fellow great apes routinely eat today may seem foreign to many of us today — such as bugs, dirt, feces and tree bark — ways to replace them with more palatable options do exist to help make optimal ancestral nutrition much more accessible and palatable for you and your family.

To get you started off on the right foot, this book also covers exactly what plant foods should be a critical part of your diet and what foods to avoid, as well as how to prepare them optimally to retain their nutritional value. It also provides creative ideas for what to eat in a day via a range of tasty meal plans, and it describes in detail how to make some delicious recipes to get you inspired during your transition.

In general, keep in mind that if you can eat plant foods as fresh and raw as possible, then this is virtually always the best way to get your nutrition, but if this is challenging for you, then eating dried fruits, seeds and nuts, and using food processing techniques like freezing and low-temperature dehydration will preserve many key nutrients and can support your journey to optimal health.

If you are reading this book, then there's a very good chance that you've already discovered the value of focusing on plant foods in your diet and are ready for a healthy change within your own life and to be a beacon of compassionate dietary change for those around you. If you're ready to eat a raw, plant-based diet like your Pliocene ancestors that is free of potentially-problematic and relatively modern agricultural products like legumes and grains, then now is the time for you to read this book and join the Pliocene Diet tribe.

If you are like most people seeking to regain or safeguard their health, you probably can't wait to celebrate the reclamation of your ancestral and compassionate birthright to the radical health and vitality our Pliocene ancestors enjoyed! You just have to start including the most nutrient-rich foods on the planet in your diet as you focus on consuming natural, raw plant foods.

CHAPTER 2: THE SCIENCE OF NUTRITION

Before getting into the details of how and why to follow a diet that your pre-human ancestors would have been comfortable eating way back in the Pliocene Epoch that dated from 5.333 million to 2.58 million years before the present time, it first makes sense to introduce the science of nutrition. This will provide you with a basic understanding of what modern-day humans need to eat to be healthy and why some diets tend to be more or less healthy for humans than others.

Macronutrients and Micronutrients

In the science of nutrition, the term "macronutrient" refers to the three main types of food required in large amounts in a particular species' diet, which are proteins, fats and carbohydrates, and from which energy can be derived. In contrast, micronutrients refer to dietary components that are required in smaller amounts for optimal health, and they include vitamins, minerals and phytochemicals.

Phytochemicals are biologically-active substances that come from plants and may have an impact on health. Such bioactive chemicals typically act as natural pesticides that plants use to protect themselves from herbivorous creatures. Within a diet, phytochemicals may boost the activity or production of enzymes. This can help prevent heart disease and stroke, as well as block carcinogens and suppress the proliferation of malignant cells.

Carbohydrates

Carbohydrates or carbs are an excellent source of dietary energy and provide 4 calories per gram consumed. They are further broken down into dietary fiber, complex carbohydrates and simple sugars, while the "net carbs" in a particular food consists of the total amount of carbohydrates in a portion minus the amount of fiber. This is widely considered a more important measure of the carbohydrates in food because fiber cannot be digested by your body, so it does not raise your blood sugar levels enough to trigger an insulin response.

Insulin is the key hormone in your body that is responsible for causing the deposition of fat when blood sugar levels rise too high. Many nutritionists look at the Glycemic Index (GI) of carbohydrate-containing foods to rank them according to their effect on blood glucose levels that can prompt the release of insulin when too high. Foods that have a low GI value of 55 or less digest more slowly in your body, so when their carbohydrates are absorbed and metabolized, they cause a slower rise in blood glucose to lower levels that in turn reduce insulin production and hence fat deposition.

Proteins

When it comes to proteins, they are essential nutrients for humans because they help build body tissue, although consuming excessive amounts can acidify the human body and lead to breakdown and disease. Proteins can also serve as a source of energy, providing 4 calories per gram like carbohydrates. What distinguishes a protein is that it is composed of building blocks called amino acids linked together in a particular order by peptide bonds. When humans digest proteins, they are broken down by stomach acids and digestive enzymes into smaller polypeptide chains that are easier for the body to absorb essential amino acids from.

An essential amino acid is one of nine that cannot be synthesized by the human body and that humans therefore need to get from their diet to prevent protein deficiency. For adults, they consist of histidine, isoleucine, lysine, leucine, methionine, phenylalanine, threonine, tryptophan and valine, although histidine is synthesized in children. Humans can also make five amino acids, specifically alanine, asparagine, aspartic acid, glutamic acid and serine. In certain people, the synthesis of some amino acids can be limited by physiological pathologies, so they become essential to obtain from their diet. These amino acids include arginine, cysteine, glutamine, glycine, proline and tyrosine.

Fats

Dietary fats are a possible source of energy and provide 9 calories per gram, which is over twice that provided by carbs and proteins. Fats are categorized as saturated, mono-unsaturated and poly-unsaturated fats. The degree of saturation of a fat molecule depends on how many double bonds are formed in its hydrocarbon chain. The fewer double bonds involved, the straighter the fat molecules are and the more they can stack together, so the more solid the fat becomes.

That explains why a highly-saturated fat like coconut oil is typically solid at room temperature, while a largely unsaturated fat like olive oil is typically a liquid. Heating will tend to liquefy a saturated fat because heat starts the fat molecules vibrating and enough heat will eventually cause the fat to melt as the molecules separate from each other into a liquid state.

Humans Should Restrict Their Intake of Saturated Fats and Cholesterol

All animal products contain a lipoprotein called cholesterol that comes in low-density and high-density forms that are known as LDL (low-density lipoprotein) and HDL (high-density lipoprotein) cholesterol respectively. HDL cholesterol is sometimes called "good" cholesterol because it picks up excess cholesterol circulating in your blood and takes it to your liver to be broken down and removed from your body.

While HDL cholesterol is currently not considered problematic, LDL cholesterol is widely thought among researchers and cardiologists to contribute to vascular disorders like heart disease by forming arterial plaque that accumulates on and therefore hardens and narrows your arteries wherever your blood circulates in your body.

Plaque deposits cause poor circulation that can result in blood clots, and they can also break off and clog arteries, both of which can lead to heart attacks and strokes that can be fatal. Arterial plaque can also cause high blood pressure by preventing hardened arteries from contracting and expanding naturally as blood volume fluctuates.

Most importantly, the more saturated fats you consume, the more your body makes unhealthy LDL cholesterol. Many nutritionists therefore consider keeping saturated fat intake low to be more important to managing your blood LDL cholesterol level than minimizing the amount of cholesterol you obtain from foods.

Furthermore, since humans manufacture all the cholesterol they need, the human diet has no need to include any added cholesterol whatsoever. Most dietary experts now agree that the healthiest human diet should also be low in saturated fats so that the body does not make as much problematic LDL cholesterol.

Since cholesterol is only found in animal products, this means the optimal human diet should consist exclusively of plant-derived foods that also contain low levels of saturated fat.

The Science Highlights the Dangers of Consuming Animal Products

Dr. Michael Greger is a medical doctor who has spent much of his career studying and raising awareness about the adverse impact of animal products on human health. He has collected some of his science-based research into his best-selling book "How Not to Die: Discover the Foods Scientifically Proven to Prevent and Reverse Disease"[2], and he has also published such research on his educational website NutritionFact.org[3] and his extensive YouTube channel.[4] Dr. Greger notes that although animal products are a central part of the standard American diet, they are linked to a range of unhealthy conditions in the scientific literature.

In fact, Dr. Greger shows in his aforementioned book that consuming animal products increases your chances of dying from 14 out of the 15 leading causes of death in the United States, with the lone exception being accidents. Although this tragic reality is still unknown to many people who still persist in consuming animal products, it was becoming evident to scientists and medical researchers as early as 1907 when the New York Times covered a study that indicated the increased consumption of animal-derived foods was a major factor in the 4,600 cancer cases it reviewed.

Furthermore, the massive Cornell-Oxford-China study conducted in the 1970s and '80s showed that even small amounts of food derived from animals were associated with a notable increase in the risk of suffering from certain

[2] https://www.amazon.com/How-Not-Die-Discover-Scientifically/dp/1250066115/

[3] https://nutritionfacts.org/

[4] https://www.youtube.com/channel/UCddn8dUxYdgJz3Qr5mjADtA

chronic diseases. That milestone led to the publication in 2008 of the classic book by China Study leader Dr. Caldwell Esselstyn called "Prevent and Reverse Heart Disease: The Revolutionary, Scientifically Proven, Nutrition-Based Cure" which actively promoted using a plant-based diet to treat America's #1 killer.

Diets rich in animal foods have also been linked in many studies to a higher risk for heart disease and cancer mortality. Consuming animal food is additionally associated with a greater risk of being overweight, which might be related to the fact that the regular consumption of animal foods and poor-quality junk foods high in fat calories can dull our brain's pleasure center sufficiently that we tend to overeat.

One study's researchers noted improvement in key health measures in people who followed a diet free of animal products for just 21 days. Another study showed that putting Parkinson's disease patients on a strict plant-based diet free of all animal products led to a significant reduction in their symptoms. Reducing junk food and animal product consumption for even a few weeks may help your tongue become more sensitive to fat, which can in turn make you less likely to overeat and help combat obesity.

Dr. Greger also notes that numerous peer-reviewed research studies have found links between the intake of animal products and the risks of suffering from the following diseases and adverse health conditions:

- Allergic, autoimmune and inflammatory disorders
- Cancer
- Cataracts
- Cellulite
- Dementia
- Diabetes: Type 2 diabetes, prediabetes, and gestational diabetes
- Insulin resistance
- Life-threatening reactions to E. coli toxins
- Gallstones
- Recurrent gout attacks
- Neurological diseases
- Prepuberty

- Prostatic hyperplasia
- Rheumatoid arthritis
- Declining sperm counts

He also observes that cutting back or eliminating animal product consumption in favor of increasing your intake of whole plant foods has many potential benefits shown in various studies, including the fact that this diet:

- Helps with weight control
- Slows the aging process
- Slows the growth of certain cancers
- Slows body cell death rates
- Slows the progression of rheumatoid arthritis, cancer, diabetes and heart disease
- Reduces insulin sensitivity
- Increases the chances for breast cancer survival
- Increases antioxidant intake
- Increases the intake of fiber
- Helps improve mood
- Avoids inflammation caused by endotoxemia
- Helps lower LDL cholesterol levels
- Helps manage mental health conditions
- Slows the shrinking of muscle mass as a person ages
- Decreases oxidative stress
- Increases the intake of phytate, an anticarcinogen
- Boosts levels of serotonin
- Helps treat acne

According to Dr. Greger, animal products also contain a number of substances notably unhealthy for humans that occur naturally, are added to animal feed or are accumulated from the toxic environment farmed animals are generally kept in. These include:

- AGEs
- Arachidonic acid
- Arsenic
- Cadmium
- DDT and dioxins

- Organochlorine pollutants
- Phosphates
- Pollutants, including highly toxic mercury, especially from fish products
- Steroid hormones

Government-Promoted Dietary Policies and Subsidies Need to Change

The official policies of various governments as they relate to animal products have also been overly favorable, which has become controversial due to the notable harm it causes to their citizens. Promoting animal product consumption has tragically become the norm largely due to active lobbying by the powerful profit-hungry industries that promote, sell or produce animal-derived foods for human consumption. A notable example of such deeply-flawed nutritional policies in the United States is the official Dietary Guidelines and those set by the USDA.

As a result of the overwhelming scientific evidence in favor of a whole foods plant-based diet for humans, some health advocates have suggested that reducing government subsidies would be one sensible way to reduce their consumption by humans. In the U.S., only animal products and plant feed crops intended for farmed animals are heavily subsidized by the government which helps make animal food products so artificially cheap in the country. This contributes to widespread epidemic of chronic diseases like heart disease, cancer, obesity and Type II diabetes.

The science is now very clear that eliminating these subsidies would allow prices for unhealthy food items to increase, thereby reducing consumption and notably improving the health of the human population. Government subsidy money could then flow toward making whole plant foods that actually promote human health more affordable and universally available. Since farming animal products is also very wasteful of human edible food, this shift could free up substantial food supplies to feed hungry humans around the world and make starvation among our species a thing of the past.

CHAPTER 3: ANCESTRAL VS. MODERN DIETS

The phrase "ancestral diet" includes numerous diets that are based on what their various proponents claim were the likely eating patterns of ancient humans and/or their hominid ancestors.

Furthermore, the term "hominids" refers to a primate of a family called Hominidae that includes humans, their extinct ancestors known from the fossil record, and also at least some of the other great apes. Existing great apes include humans, gorillas, orangutans, chimpanzees and bonobos.

The Physiological Human Diet

The theory behind eating based on the ancestral diet for your species is that you will be healthier when eating foods that your body is best adapted for on a physiological level. This brings up another key scientific concept when it comes to discussing ancestral diets known as a "physiological diet", which is the way of eating dictated by a creature's physiology, including its innate ability to obtain and digest certain foods based upon its natural endowments.

The image shown on the following page illustrates how humans measure up to other species in terms of their physiological diet. As you will note from that chart, humans clearly have no notable predatory physical characteristics, digestive apparatus or other adaptations to consume flesh, eggs or the mammary secretions of other creatures.

This set of facts has prompted many modern-day science-based observers to conclude that predation, scavenging and the subsequent consumption of animal-derived items is as unnatural for humans as it is for our other great ape cousins.

CARNIVORE	OMNIVORE	HERBIVORE	FRUGIVOROUS	HUMAN
Physiological food: meat	PF: meat and vegetables	Physiological food: herbs	PF: fruits, vegetables & nuts	PF: fruits, vegetables & nuts
4 paws with claws	4 paws with claws / hooves	4 paws with hooves	Prehensile hands and feet	Prehensile hands
Walk on 4 paws	Walk on 4 paws	Walk on 4 paws	Walks on 4 paws/ upright	Walks upright
Mouth opening: Large	Mouth opening: Large	Mouth opening: Small	Mouth opening: Small / M	Mouth opening: Small
Great sharp fangs	Great sharp fangs	Rudimentary, blunt canines	Canines for defense	Rudimentary, blunt canines
Short and pointed incisors	Short and pointed incisors	Big and flattened incisors	Big and flattened incisors	Big and flattened incisors
Blade shaped molars	Blade shaped/crushing molars	Flattened & strong molars	Flattened molars	Flattened molars
Lower jaw embedded inside of the top; no lateral or forward mobility	Lower jaw embedded inside of the top; no lateral or forward mobility / minimal	Upper jaw sits on the bottom; great lateral and forward mobility	Upper jaw sits on the bottom; great lateral and forward mobility	Upper jaw sits on the bottom; great lateral and forward mobility
Shear; swallow w/o chewing	Shear & swallow / crushing	No shear; chew much	No shear; chew their food	No shear; chew their food
Small salivary glands	Small salivary glands	Big salivary glands	Big salivary glands	Big salivary glands
Acid saliva without ptyalin	Acid saliva without ptyalin	Alkaline saliva with ptyalin	Alkaline saliva with ptyalin	Alkaline saliva with ptyalin
Acid urine	Acid urine	Alkaline urine	Alkaline urine	Alkaline urine
Renal secretion of uricase	Renal secretion of uricase	Not secrete uricase	Not secrete uricase	Not secrete uricase
Strong Hydrochloric acid	Strong Hydrochloric acid	Weak Hydrochloric acid	Weak Hydrochloric acid	Weak Hydrochloric acid
Does not require fiber to stimulate peristalsis	Does not require fiber to stimulate peristalsis	Require fiber to stimulate peristalsis	Require fiber to stimulate peristalsis	Require fiber to stimulate peristalsis
Metabolize large amount of cholesterol and vitamin A	Metabolize large amount of cholesterol and vitamin A	Metabolize small amount of cholesterol and vitamin A	Metabolize small amount of cholesterol and vitamin A	Metabolize small amount of cholesterol and vitamin A
Sweat glands in the paws; gasp to cool the blood	Sweat glands in whole body	Sweat glands in whole body	Sweat glands in whole body	Sweat glands in whole body
Intestine from 1.5 to 3 times body length	Intestine 3 times body length	Intestine 20 times body length	Intestine 9 times body length	Intestine 9 times body length
Colon short smooth alkaline	Colon short smooth alkaline	Colon long complex acid	Colon long sacculated acid	Colon long sacculated acid
Not metabolize cellulose	Not metabolize cellulose	Metabolize cellulose	Not metabolize cellulose	Not metabolize cellulose
Complete digestion 2 to 4 hs	Complete digestion 6 to 10 hs	Complete digestion 24 to 48 hs	Complete digestion 12 to 18 hs	Complete digestion 12 to 18 hs

A physiological analysis of humans versus carnivores, omnivores, herbivores and frugivores.

We do not have to believe the scientists when thinking about this topic though, since any human can easily look at their own body for further physiological evidence to ascertain that they were never naturally adapted to catch, kill and consume other creatures. Humans have no sharp and pointy teeth to rip flesh with, and no big sharp claws or ability to run very fast to catch prey. They also typically lack the low stomach pH and short digestive system to speed up the digestion of meat protein and saturated fats that predators have, nor do they have anything else that identifies them as a physiological carnivore or even omnivore.

Another major issue with most modern human diets is that they include the mammary secretions of non-human animals. The females of all mammalian species produce milk of a specific type as food intended just for their young, not for members of any other species or even for adults of their own species. Since the consumption of this milk also generally concludes upon weaning for a particular non-human species, it does not naturally continue into adolescence or adulthood.

Humans consuming the milk of another species when they are infants without teeth might be justifiable as a matter of survival if their own mother or a human wet nurse were unable to provide milk for them, but them doing so past the age of weaning is notably unnatural behavior since no other species on Earth does something this strange. This dietary error also tends to increase the risk of obesity and vascular diseases in adult humans due to the high cholesterol and saturated fat intake associated with whole milk or dairy product consumption.

Why Humans Should be Eating Plants

The overwhelming conclusion to be drawn from scientifically-derived evidence like that presented previously is that humans are best adapted to consuming an alkalizing frugivorous diet that consists mainly of fruits, vegetables, herbs, nuts and seeds after weaning from their own mothers' milk, just like our closest cousins among the other great apes.

Basically, our digestive physiology and our circulatory system that evolved during the Pliocene Epoch is best suited for eating plants. Our natural physiology never adapted to allow us to thrive while consuming the animal foods provided by the relatively modern man-made technology of killing with weapons or by captive bolt guns in a slaughterhouse. Neither are humans well suited to consuming products from the outrageously cruel, disease-ridden and overcrowded animal factory farms that facilitate widespread flesh, dairy and egg product consumption by humans in the modern era.

While developing the technology to provide flesh foods to hungry hominids may have initially promoted our survival as a species when our ancestors' forest homes turned into plains as a result of climate change, it unfortunately left us divorced from our most natural and healthiest ancestral diet that evolved during the Pliocene epoch and was based almost exclusively on plant foods. This is the same healthful diet rich in plant foods that modern-day great apes like gorillas, bonobos and orangutans still follow in their natural forest environments.

Although humans may survive for some time on an omnivorous diet, they stand a notably lower chance on average of thriving well into old age on one compared to those following a well-balanced, whole foods plant-based diet that our physiology is best adapted for. Numerous studies have shown that those following a plant-based diet are slimmer and healthier on average, and they also have a statistically significant lower chance of dying from 14 of the leading 15 causes of death in the U.S., with the lone exception being accidents.

Another common benefit of following an ancestral diet is that you will eventually attain a slim bodyweight best suited for avoiding predators and long-term survival in general if the diet is followed for a sufficient length of time. While most obese people do lose weight on ancestral diets, they might also develop a vitamin or mineral deficiency[5] if they do not eat a sufficient quantity of calories and/or if they fail to consume a suitable range of raw plant-derived foods that such nutrients abound in.

This means it is generally important to follow the science-based guidance in this book and/or consult with your doctor or a qualified nutritionist before starting any new ancestral diet to make sure your nutritional bases are covered, that you are taking any necessary supplements, and that the ancestral diet is suitable for your present health condition.

---

[5] "The Gale Encyclopedia of Diets: A Guide to Health and Nutrition"; Jacqueline L. Longe, 2008.

Foraging for Food

In general, foraging means searching widely for food growing wild, such as uncultivated edible plants, mushrooms, herbs and fruits. Foraging is something practiced instinctively and naturally by many different species of animal. For our hominid ancestors, foraging meant looking around, digging, rummaging about, and picking plant foods that they knew from experience and tradition generally fell within the range of foods that were suitable for them to eat because they were both digestible and non-toxic.

Humans are especially fortunate in their ancestral biological role as plant-eaters because they can consume such a wide variety of plants. In fact, of the estimated 400,000 species of plants on Earth, it is thought by researchers like John Warren, author of <u>The Nature of Crops: How We Came to Eat the Plants We Do</u> [6], that roughly 300,000 plant species are edible by humans, although we presently only cultivate about 200 of them for food.

Furthermore, while many foraged plant foods can be eaten directly after harvesting, certain foraged food items contain defensive poisons or physical barriers, so they need to be prepared in specific ways to make them less toxic, more nutritious and/or more digestible. Over the millennia, humans have evolved various ways to enhance the edibility of certain raw plant foods by soaking, sprouting and/or marinating them, for example.

In the context of this book, foraging is what our hominid ancestors generally did to find edible plant foods before they invented and took up weapons to begin scavenging, hunting and fishing other animals to help supplement their diet. Foraging also excludes more modern ways of obtaining flesh or dairy products from farmed domesticated animals, such as shepherding, ranching or intensive industrial animal farming in concentrated animal feeding operations or CAFOs which are also often called factory farms.

Our hominid ancestors must have understood that foraging for wild food was a delightful way to experience the natural world. Today, we can still engage in that instinctive activity to connect with something primal and prehistoric within ourselves. In many ways, foraging for food presents a

---

[6] https://www.amazon.com/Nature-Crops-How-Came-Plants/dp/1780645090

considerably healthier and more nutritious alternative to consuming the processed foods found at most modern grocery stores.

Food foraged from the wild is considerably richer in essential vitamins and minerals and does not have any toxic pesticides or fertilizer residues. Also, the very act of foraging provides us with healthy exercise in a natural setting and the opportunity to breathe fresh air. In fact, foraging combines the best aspects of both hiking and organic gardening!

Before starting your own excursion into the exciting world of wild food foraging, you will want to educate yourself about some basic rules that will make your foraging activities both safe and sustainable. The first and most sensible rule of foraging is to avoid eating anything you are not absolutely sure you have correctly identified as edible. Some plants are poisonous, so you need to learn to avoid them. Consulting with experts on plant identification and carrying an edible food guide with you when foraging can help in this regard.

Secondly, while Nature is resilient, you can seriously traumatize an ecosystem by overharvesting its plants. By harvesting wild-growing plant foods as sustainably as possible, you will be able to harvest more edible plants from the same location in the coming years, which will ultimately make foraging so much easier for you. In addition to avoiding over-harvesting, sustainable harvesting means you want to avoid killing the food plant if at all possible. You should also refrain from harming any protected and/or endangered species, and you should not harvest more food than you will actually use.

Third, make sure the area you intend to forage in is not contaminated. Poisoning can result from the presence of heavy metals in the soil, as well as from man-made toxins released by chemical manufacturing plants and military bases. Animal agriculture facilities can also pollute nearby waterways with manure and cause toxic algae blooms.

Finally, make sure that foraging in a particular area is legal. Check for no trespassing signs if you do not have the property owner's permission to forage in a particular private location. Also, make sure to review any park regulations relevant to foraging first if you intend to harvest food plants in a public park.

An increasingly popular alternative to foraging in the wild is to create your very own food forest, as described further in my book "The Food Forest Guide".[7] This involves planting and cultivating a variety of food-bearing trees and edible plants in your own garden as part of the landscaping process. You can then not only enjoy foraging in your own backyard, but you will have a food source at home you can fall back on to increase your family's resilience in times of financial difficulty or if a disaster occurs that disrupts the food supply in your area.

---

[7] https://www.amazon.com/Food-Forest-Guide-Cultivate-Landscape/dp/B0CKW96GW1

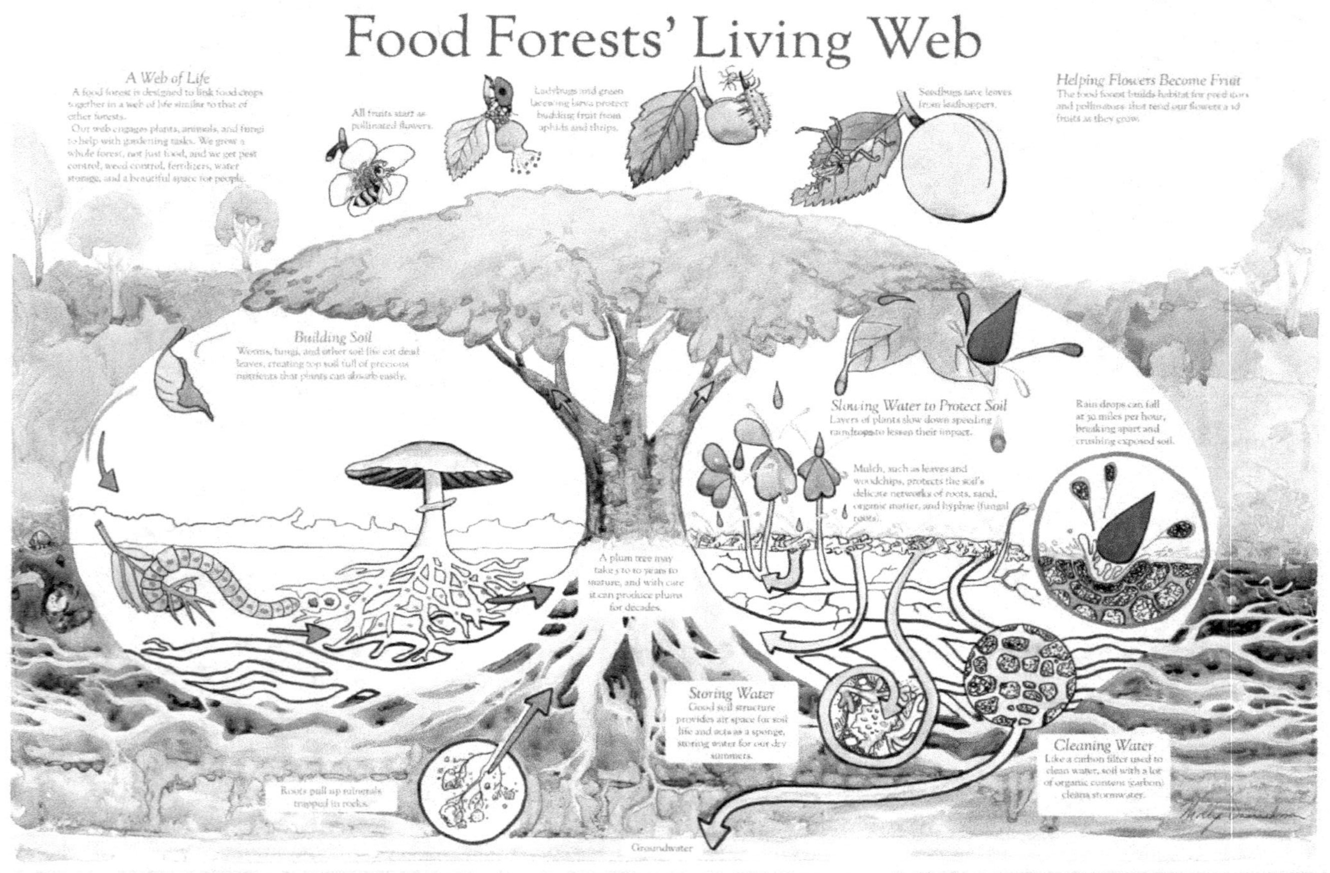

How an ideal food forest operates to create a living web and habitat that can also feed you.

The Paleolithic Diet Theory

In recent years, considerable attention has focused on the so-called Paleolithic or Paleo ancestral diet that arose in hominids and then humans during the period that stretched from around 2.58 million years ago, all the way up until around 10,000 years before the present time (BP). The theory behind Paleo eating is that this pre-historical era covered the time when humans had evolved to their present genetic state but had not yet started the now-widespread plant and animal agricultural practices modern food is generally derived from.

According to a study published in 2006 by S. Boyd Eton in The Proceedings of the Nutrition Society[8] a typical Paleolithic ancestral human diet dating from 50-100,000 years ago had an estimated 35 percent of its dietary calories coming from fats. Regarding fat intake types, the level of saturated fats in the Paleo ancestral diet contributed roughly 7.5% of calories, while harmful trans-fatty acids were only present in tiny amounts and the level of polyunsaturated fat intake was high. Furthermore, the ratio of Omega−6 to Omega−3 fatty acids approached a reasonably healthy 2 to 1 ratio compared to the much higher 10 to 1 ratio seen on average today in many modern Western diets. Keeping trans fatty acids to a minimum and a low Omega 6 to Omega 3 ratio in your diet are both healthful practices.

An additional 35 percent of dietary calories came from carbohydrates, while the last 30 percent of dietary calories came from protein. Furthermore, around 50 percent of the carbohydrate intake in Paleolithic ancestral human diets came from uncultivated raw fruits and vegetables, compared with the modern Standard American Diet which only averages around 16 percent from whole fruit and vegetable sources. Also, the fiber content of the ancestral diet was high and more than adequate for health, probably averaging in the region of 100 grams per day. Studies have shown that eating more plant fiber and raw plant foods tends to improve human health and reduce obesity.

In addition, the relatively high intake of fresh fruits and vegetables in ancestral diets combined with the minimal intake of grains, legumes, animal

---

[8] Eaton, S. (2006). The ancestral human diet: What was it and should it be a paradigm for contemporary nutrition? *Proceedings of the Nutrition Society, 65*(1), 1-6. doi:10.1079/PNS2005471

proteins and dairy products, typically resulted in an alkalinizing or base-yielding diet that supports good human health and delays aging. This contrasts notably with the heavily acid-forming diets now common in Western countries containing substantial amounts of cooked and processed plant foods, along with the high-protein animal-derived foods that promote an acidic body condition implicated in causing chronic diseases and early aging.

With respect to sugars, raw honey only comprised probably 2 to 3 percent of our Paleolithic ancestors' energy intake, compared with the much higher percentage of their energy intake that many modern humans get from problematic highly-processed sweeteners like sucrose and high fructose corn syrup.

While fructose generally comes from fruits that are part of our healthiest ancestral dietary pattern, note that sucrose is generally derived from a grass-family plant (the sugar cane) and from a starchy root vegetable (beets). Since neither class of plant is part of any ancestral diets for humans (other than perhaps in a desperate survival situation involving starvation), sucrose is just not suitable for humans, and especially not in its refined form of table sugar. Furthermore, sucrose competes with the precious vitamin C that boosts our immune systems, making it a potent and even deadly anti-nutrient.

Naturally derived fructose from fruit sources is not associated with the same negative health outcomes as sucrose. Fruit also does not contain the same combination of glucose and fructose that the widely used artificial ingredient high fructose corn syrup does. Also, the health benefits of eating fruit outweigh any potential negative effects of its natural fructose, given the high fiber content and vitamins, minerals, and antioxidants found in fruit. [9]

The content of legume-bearing anti-cancer nutrients like phytates in Paleolithic diets was also quite low, while the intake of micronutrients like vitamins, minerals and phytochemicals was typically 1.5 to 8 times that of those following modern Western diets.

When it comes to the consumption of sodium, Paleolithic diets contained

---

[9] Stricker S, Rudloff S, Geier A, Steveling A, Roeb E, Zimmer KP. Fructose Consumption-Free Sugars and Their Health Effects. Dtsch Arztebl Int. 2021 Feb 5;118(5):71-78. doi: 10.3238/arztebl.m2021.0010. PMID: 33785129; PMCID: PMC8188419. Retrieved from: https://pubmed.ncbi.nlm.nih.gov/33785129/

generally less than 1 gram per day, which was much less than the consumption of potassium. This stands in marked contrast to today's high-sodium diets that typically involve the addition of table salt (sodium chloride) to highly-processed prepared food, as well as during cooking and at the table. This excessive salting of food also notably exceeds the amount of potassium consumed to an unhealthy degree.

In addition, keeping table salt intake low tends to contribute to better vascular health due to its deadly blood pressure increasing effect when arterial hardening is present. The World Health Organization[10] estimates that 2.5 million human deaths could be prevented if human salt consumption was reduced to less than the 5 grams per day amount that it recommends.

Where Paleo Diets Fail

Unfortunately for the Paleo dietary theory, the Paleolithic or Stone Age era started precisely when early hominids began using stone tools as weapons and processing tools that facilitated scavenging, hunting, and the unnatural consumption of animal flesh that was previously not practical for them with their natural physical adaptations.

Since cooking also began in the Paleolithic era, the Paleo diet includes cooked foods that lack vital nutrients destroyed by heat, such as vitamin C that boosts your immune system and the B vitamins that are essential for maintaining healthy energy levels and nervous systems in humans. The ancestral diet that hominids used tools and fire to consume in the Paleo era does not therefore feature the healthier raw plant foods that dominated their diet during the preceding Pliocene epoch. The Pliocene diet is thus far superior to the later Paleo diet because it is generally fully raw and devoid of animal products, other than including human breast milk for babies until the age of their weaning.

Furthermore, while the Paleo diet has some positives relative to the notably poor and highly-processed diet many humans presently consume, it lacks the long term health benefits since it is just too high in fat calories, cholesterol, and starch humans. Accordingly, following the fat-heavy Paleo

---

[10] https://www.who.int/news-room/fact-sheets/detail/salt-reduction

diet can lead to obesity, insulin resistance, Type II diabetes and the serious vascular diseases that inhibit circulation and result in high blood pressure, impotence, and the deadly heart attacks and strokes that presently kill more humans in the US than any other cause.

Also, since the Paleo diet is too high in acid-forming proteins from flesh and includes cooked plant foods that are also acid-forming, following the Paleo diet can result in an overly acidic body pH. This unhealthy condition breaks down tissues causing premature aging and promotes deadly chronic diseases like certain cancers that tend to thrive and advance in acidic body conditions.

Why The Pliocene Diet is Vastly Superior to The Paleo Diet

The Pliocene epoch of human evolution stretched from 5.333 million to 2.58 million years before the present time, and it featured hominids who were the direct line ancestors of modern humans. They did not use cutting tools or weapons so they generally did not hunt or scavenge, and they foraged for food rather than farming it so they did not consume grains or legumes to any significant degree. They also typically lived in forests and primarily consumed plants, fruits, nuts and seeds in their raw natural state.

The ancestral Pliocene diet was thus based almost entirely on raw plant-derived foods with only trivial amounts of nutrients obtained from insects and other sources. The far more natural Pliocene ancestral diet that preceded the Paleo dietary pattern thus lacks all of the Paleo diet's shortcomings while retaining all of its benefits for modern humans since plant-based diets have a long science-based history of being much healthier for humans to consume overall than meat-heavy diets.

As further proof of the Pliocene diet's superiority to Paleo, it is exactly the same sort of natural, raw plant-based diet currently followed in the wild by our existing great ape cousins the chimpanzees, bonobos and orangutans. This healthier ancestral diet has clearly passed the test of being consumed for millennia by our existing hominid family and our ancestors.

The Pliocene diet is not only more natural for humans than the Paleo diet, but it is notably lower in deadly artery-clogging saturated fats and cholesterol. In fact, the Pliocene diet our ancestors ate likely had a macronutrient calorie ratio closer to the 10 percent protein, 10 percent fat and 80 percent carbohydrates (including fiber) ratio that experts currently considered healthiest for humans, including medical doctors with nutritional expertise like Dr. Douglas Graham, Author of The 80-10-10 Diet.[11]

Rather than erroneously focusing on the more recent Paleo ancestral diet that was facilitated by obviously unnatural weaponry, tools and cooking, while being unnecessarily tainted by fat, cholesterol and protein-laden animal products that humans really have no business eating other than in a desperate survival situation, it makes far more sense to go back to what our relatively peaceful Pliocene ancestors ate. This is especially true if you really want to stay healthy, free from chronic disease and trim as you age gracefully so that you can thrive well into your golden years and cultivate the good health needed to enjoy them.

---

[11] https://www.amazon.com/80-10-Diet/dp/1893831248/

CHAPTER 4: PLIOCENE DIET PRINCIPLES

In a nutshell, the Pliocene Diet is all about eating only those natural foods that people living in the pre-agricultural age could have eaten safely before fire was used for cooking, weapons were crafted for killing and tools were made for cutting flesh. Foods approved for those on the Pliocene Diet are therefore entirely derived from plants, although many Pliocene dieters also often exclude agricultural seeds like grains and legumes. Suitable plant foods are also not processed or packaged, nor are they ever cooked since that practice did not become common until Paleolithic times around 2 million years ago, according to Richard Wrangham, author of Catching Fire: How Cooking Made Us Human. [12]

Raw Versus Cooked

Although plant foods can generally be consumed raw for optimal nutrition, cooking was largely necessary in the Paleolithic era as a way for early humans to consume bacteria-infested flesh and other animal products safely without getting sick from that unnatural behavior they participated in.

Since cooking plant foods notably reduces their nutritional value by destroying the especially sensitive C and B vitamins and by denaturing enzymes that assist in food digestion, it should ideally be avoided entirely while on the Pliocene Diet. This means keeping the temperature of your food below that of the hot sun, which would be around 117 degrees Fahrenheit. Dehydration of food in the sun or in a dehydrator set at or below that maximum temperature is permissible on the Pliocene Diet. This can assist you in creating different and firmer food textures, such as those found in crackers, nut loaves, nut patties, and Essene breads.

---

[12] http://www.amazon.com/Catching-Fire-Cooking-Made-Human/dp/0465020410/

A major advantage of strictly following the Pliocene Diet is that it has a net dietary alkaline load that promotes good health and slows aging. The fact that the diet is entirely plant-based and is naturally low in calories also means that it reduces the risk of chronic diseases and deadly health events associated with animal product consumption, including heart disease, strokes, some cancers, obesity and diabetes.

Pliocene Diet-approved foods therefore do not include animal products or cooked items. They also tend to have the following characteristics in common:

- Low in fat
- No cholesterol
- Low in calories
- Low score on the glycemic index
- High in fiber
- Low in sodium
- High in vitamins, minerals, antioxidants and plant phytochemicals.

In terms of a target macronutrient ratio, Pliocene Dieters should aim to get roughly 10% of their calories from fats, 10% from proteins and 80% from carbohydrates. Using a nutritional app on your cell phone or a website like Cronometer.com can help you watch your caloric intake while making sure the food choices you make while on your unique Pliocene Diet covers all of your macronutrient and micronutrient bases.

With respect to the food types consumed on the ideal Pliocene Diet that is fruit-based or "frugivorous" in nature, foods should consist of roughly 50% fruits, 40% greens and 10% nuts, seeds, good fats like avocadoes and coconuts, and vegetables. This is very similar to the natural dietary ratios that our close genetic relatives the peaceful bonobos might consume in the modern era.

Keep in mind that since humans do require tiny amounts of Vitamin B12, which is produced by microbes, either a supplement should be taken periodically or sources like nutritional yeast should be consumed regularly. Also, if you do not get enough Vitamin D3 from natural sunlight exposure on your skin, then you can take a D3 supplement derived from lichen since the Vitamin D2 you can obtain from mushrooms may not be sufficient for your nutritional needs.

Using Raw Fruit and Salads to Keep Your Digestive Tract Healthy

The true ancestral diet eaten when the human digestive tract was evolved to its current general state was largely based on the consumption of raw fruit and other plant foods, as was seen among hominids in the Pliocene Era. This same diet is also currently seen among present day great apes like chimpanzees, bonobos and orangutans to further demonstrate this point.

Since humans remain physiologically best suited to eating fruit, it should come as no surprise that eating fruit helps us maintain a healthy digestive system. Fruit does not cause intestinal problems, and it does not block intestines with accumulated waste that can lead to ulcers, impacted feces and worse.

The modern animal product heavy diet that some humans consume generates high amounts of acidity in the body that in turn creates corrosion in the digestive tract. Animal flesh is largely composed of amino acids and saturated fats, and consuming such inappropriate foods that the human body cannot process or assimilate properly, and which contain high amounts of sticky saturated fats and and have a chemistry heavy on the acidic side promotes the breakdown of intestinal walls and harms digestive organs like the pancreas and gallbladder.

Also, when the hair-like villi of the small intestines become clogged with the saturated fat from animal products that plasters the walls of the small intestine, this blocks the nutrients from your food from entering into your cells and leads to the malabsorption of essential vitamins and minerals. The end result of this problem is nutrient deficiency, poor overall health and possibly even overeating in order to get the nutrients your body craves.

Consuming cooked starches, proteins and fats of all kinds also creates ulcerations in the intestines over time. Such a diet also leads to the accumulation of wastes in the large intestine or colon that cannot be properly eliminated. This in turn creates a breeding ground for parasites, fungus and yeasts that also block the flow of waste removal and can lead to chronic constipation.

In contrast, consuming fruit does not have this effect, and neither does the consumption of non-starchy vegetables. Furthermore, fruit cleans the colon more effectively because the intestinal transit time of fruit is fast and fruit is astringent by nature. Fruits both cleanse the colon and help remove impacted feces from it.

Eating a lot of tough plant fiber matter can be hard on the human digestion too because heavy cellulose fiber like that found in grass or wood just isn't appropriate for humans either. As a great ape, remember that you're a member of an animal species and your species has a specific physiological diet it is adapted to consume, just like any other species.

Cows and other herbivorous species have large grinding teeth and produce an enzyme called cellulase that is used to break down the cellulose fibers in grass. Some of them also have multiple stomachs that allow bacterial fermentation to help with that breakdown process and let them properly digest and assimilate tough plant matter and fibers.

Humans do not produce that cellulase enzyme, and they have rather small jaws and teeth and a single stomach. This means they are far more suited for a frugivorous diet heavy in fruit, just like the other existing great apes that humans share a common ancestor with.

Fruit is naturally alkalinizing when ripe, and it treats the colon gently. Fruit also helps the kidneys filter the lymphatic system that the intestines are connected to, and eating fruit facilitates the drainage of interstitial debris within the colon.

Some people may notice that eating significant amounts of fruit can initially expose pain and create discomfort, especially if digestive ulceration already exists. This occurs because waste water accumulates in the colon, and fruit is naturally astringent so it will loosen intestinal plaques. Fruit can also ferment if digestion is slowed down by the consumption of constipating foods like starches and animal proteins. This can create gases, discomfort and even pain in the process.

Furthermore, if you have damaged your colon by eating acidifying foods like cooked foods and animal products, then mucus and even ulcers can form as a result. Consuming any type of fiber can then exacerbate the problem and cause discomfort. Fruit is fibrous and astringent, which can irritate the colon while on a fruit diet while the colon regenerates.

This explains why a juice fast focused detox period of several days until intestinal inflammation goes down makes sense. You can then start adding fruit once the intestines have healed enough to tolerate fruit fibers. It also helps afterwards to practice intermittent fasting regularly for 16-18 hours each day to encourage your kidneys to filter out so that your intestines can drain the acids that have accumulated in them.

Once your intestines have healed, your body will then enter the regenerative process when hydrated and kept alkaline with a high fruit diet. You need to stop consuming the unhealthy diet high in cooked foods and animal products that breaks down your organs, intestines and endocrine glands since processed foods, too much protein and animal fluids create excessive mucus and acidity in the body. While acids cause ulceration, an excess of mucus results in stagnation, congestion and constipation that blocks your body's natural toxin elimination pathways and reduces the nutrition you obtain from food.

Admittedly, agricultural foods are not the same now as they were when our ancestors once ate wild foods, and fruit is often harvested without ripening in the modern era. Despite lower quality fruit, many people have successfully repaired their damaged gastrointestinal tracts by eating the fruit currently available. Switching to organic fruit can also lower the amount of toxins ingested and improve the nutrition they provide.

For detoxification, fruit remains essential for regenerating deep tissues so that you can possibly start adding other foods back to your diet in future. With that noted, those suffering from chronic intestinal conditions should follow a diet strictly focused on fruits with an occasional green salad if they can tolerate the heavier fiber since that is the best way to promote faster gut healing.

Also, at the beginning of the focused detox period, you should avoid eating whole citrus fruit if you have ulcers in your intestines. It is better to instead stick to watery fruits like melons and semi acid fruits like strawberries, apples, apricots, blackberries, raspberries, blueberries, kiwi, guava, peaches, pears, plums, cherries and mangoes. Many people benefit from taking a break from eating altogether by just drinking fruit and vegetable juices and simple liquids until their internal inflammation goes down to to the point where they can tolerate whole fruits.

A diet of cooked plant foods will not extract sulfur, biofilms and mucoid plaque effectively, but fruit juice and even whole fruit will help loosen it. The fiber in salads and fruits like pineapple can act as a broom for the colon, but you shouldn't eat rough fibers or highly acidic fruit if you suffer from ulcerations or diverticulitis. Medicinal clays like bentonite clay can also be used as a colon cleansing tool along with psyllium husk and water while fasting.

Fruit cleans the intestines and helps them drain, as well as extracting the harmful acids and preventing dehydration. Fruits also assist in removing the buildup of waste from the body and leave it both hydrated and alkalinized. This allows the body to naturally enter into a state of self-healing. Always do your best to eat fruit that is sweet and mature for best results.

Basically, returning to your true nature by consuming a diet that you are biologically best suited to eat helps restore the health of your digestive system. Take advantage of your intuitive awareness and let your instincts guide your reasoning to enjoy a more suitable and healthful diet of raw fruits and salads.

Blood Sugar Considerations

For those considering the Pliocene Diet but concerned about blood sugar issues due to having developed insulin resistance, diabetes and/or obesity, the good news is that almost all Pliocene Diet-approved vegetables are low on the glycemic index, which is a scientific measure of how much a particular food spikes your blood sugar that then promotes the release of insulin by the pancreas to deposit that sugar as fat on your body.

When on the Pliocene Diet, the best vegetables to eat for such individuals are the non-starchy ones, while starchy fruits like bananas should only be eaten in moderation. If you need to watch your blood sugar, then non-starchy plant foods should make up the bulk of your carbohydrate intake and 35-45% of your daily calorie intake. The natural sugars they contain will be absorbed into your bloodstream more slowly than those from pure glucose, sucrose (pure table sugar) or starchy vegetables. As a result, you are unlikely to have a sudden surge in your blood sugar levels when eating according to Pliocene Diet principles.

CHAPTER 5: PLIOCENE DIET FOOD CHOICES

Although you may not like to think of food consumption as having "rules," when it comes to the Pliocene Diet, there are definitely foods that you should eat and ones you should avoid if you want to enjoy the benefits of his healthier ancestral diet.

For a quick "Eat This" and "Don't Eat This" primer so that you can quickly learn to make food choices appropriate for this dietary pattern, a quick reference guide to suitable food choices appears below.

EAT THIS

In general, the foods to eat on the Pliocene Diet will include raw fruits, greens, vegetables, nuts, seeds and some cold pressed oils, and will exclude animal products, grains, legumes and processed food. Infants can of course consume raw human breast milk until the time of their weaning.

No food should be bought canned, and vegetables should not be purchased frozen since they are generally blanched before freezing. Bottled food should also generally be avoided until it states "raw" on the label. Almonds, cashews and cacao will probably need to be bought raw online from specialty suppliers since they are usually heated before sale.

Nut and seed milks should be made at home in a blender from raw foods and water and instead of being purchased and packaged since they might be heated in that process.

Here is a list of some specific examples of raw foods suitable for Pliocene Dieters with relevant tips for each category.

Fruits:

Apple, avocado, blackberries, marionberries, papaya, peaches, plums, mango, lychee, blueberries, grapes, lemon, strawberries, watermelon, cantaloupe, pineapple, guava, lime, cranberries, raspberries, cantaloupe, honeydew melon, tangerine, figs, oranges, goji berries, grapefruit, tangerine, tomatoes, tomatillos, jackfruit and satsumas.

Tips: It is generally better to eat whole fruits for the beneficial fiber content instead of juicing them. Starchy fruits like bananas and plantains should only be eaten in moderation if you are concerned about blood sugar issues. Acidic fruits like the citrus fruits can also erode tooth enamel and should be rinsed off with water or consumption stopped entirely whenever teeth become sensitive to their acid content. Melons digest very quickly, so they should be consumed separately from other foods to avoid fermentation.

Greens, Land and Sea Vegetables, and Fungi:

Lettuce, spinach, kale, arugula, okra, bok choy, cabbage, asparagus, artichoke hearts, Brussel sprouts, celery, broccoli, zucchini, summer squash, peppers, cauliflower, eggplant, green onions and mushrooms. Seaweed and algae, like kelp, dulse, nori and spirulina.

Tips: Greens should be consumed with a source of vitamin C, like peppers, tomatoes, pineapple, goji berries or cranberries. High oxalate greens like spinach, dandelion greens, purslane, rhubarb, chard, endive, collard greens, mustard greens and beet greens should be consumed raw in moderation due to the potential for kidney stones. Nightshade relatives like eggplant, peppers and tomatoes should only be consumed in moderation by those suffering from inflammatory conditions like rheumatoid arthritis.

Culinary Herbs and Spices:

Cilantro, dill, basil, oregano, paprika, thyme, sage, parsley, rosemary, garlic, capsicum (hot pepper), ginger, turmeric, cinnamon, nutmeg, cumin, black or white pepper, cardamom, coriander seeds and mustard seeds. Moderate amounts of sea salt or Himalayan pink salt can be used for their mineral content, but you should add the salt yourself instead of buying food that contains it.

Starchy Vegetables:

Butternut squash, acorn squash, pumpkin, yams, taro root, cassava root (tapioca), carrots, sweet potatoes, Jerusalem artichokes and beets.

Tips: Since these vegetables are quite starchy and can spike blood sugar, be sure to eat them only in moderation if you're trying to lose weight and/or manage blood sugar issues arising from insulin resistance/diabetes. Also, since white, yellow and red potatoes are generally unpalatable raw, most Pliocene Dieters will prefer to avoid them.

Nuts and Seeds:

Almonds, cashews, hemp seeds, poppy seeds, cacao and coffee beans, hazelnuts, pecans, chestnuts, pistachios, brazil nuts, pili nuts, coconut, pine nuts, flax seeds, sesame seeds, pumpkin seeds, sunflower seeds, macadamia nuts, walnuts and chia seeds.

Tips: Nuts and seeds will be your main protein sources to be consumed in moderation to meet your 10% protein calorie percentage while on the Pliocene Diet. Note that high oxalate nuts like almonds, Brazil and pine nuts should be consumed moderately due to the potential for kidney stones. Also, pili nuts and coconut are high in saturated fat so they should be avoided by those concerned about insulin resistance and/or vascular disease.

Healthy Fats and Oils:

Raw tahini, cashew, almond, sunflower seed, macadamia nut and walnut butters, plus avocados, coconut and olives are good healthy fat-containing foods that can be consumed in moderation to meet your 10% fat calorie percentage while on the Pliocene Diet. Cold pressed oils like olive, walnut, flaxseed, macadamia, avocado and coconut oils, and coconut butter can also be used occasionally and in strict moderation.

Tips: Foods high in saturated fats like coconut oil, coconut flesh and coconut butter should be avoided entirely by those concerned about worsening existing issues with insulin resistance, Type II diabetes and/or vascular diseases like arteriosclerosis.

Miscellaneous Foods and Drinks:

Raw coconut aminos, raw apple cider vinegar, raw kimchi, raw sauerkraut, raw kombucha, maca, green tea, herbal teas, green raw coffee beans and raw unroasted cacao nibs.

Tips: Make your own drinks from scratch or read all labels carefully since many packaged products and drinks containing these items have been heated and/or come with refined sugar. Teas can be steeped in water warmed in the sun to keep them raw by not exposing them to excessive temperatures.

DON'T EAT THAT

In general, the foods to avoid on the Pliocene Diet include cooked foods, animal products, refined sugars, baked goods, agricultural products like grains and legumes, most oils and highly-processed junk foods. Specifically, these are the items you will want to avoid:

Meats
Fish
Dairy products, other than raw human breast milk for infants
Eggs
Cereal grains, such as wheat, oats, rye, corn, barley, sorghum, rice, etc.
Frozen vegetables since they are generally blanched prior to freezing
Cakes
Baked goods
Pastries
Legumes, such as peanuts, beans, peas, lentils, chickpeas, etc.
Peanut butter
Commercial ketchup
Overly salty foods
Table salt
Refined vegetable oils

Candy
Junk or processed foods
Fruit juices
Soft drinks
Alcohol
Refined sugar
Sweet syrups like high fructose corn syrup, corn syrup, honey, maple syrup and agave syrup. Only date syrup made from raw dates and water is acceptable.
Jams and jellies
Artificial sweeteners
Refined vegetable oils, such as soy, corn or canola oils.
Vegetable shortening (hydrogenated vegetable oil)
Palm oil

CHAPTER 6: OTHER DIETARY CONSIDERATIONS

Some people may wonder if supplements should even be necessary when on a natural ancestral eating plan best suited for human physiology like the Pliocene Diet. While the food sources suggested above may be very suitable, there remain several key changes in the way humans prefer to eat in the modern era that differ from how our hominid ancestors ate and so may suggest supplementation. One of the major changes is the widespread practice of washing and sterilizing food. This essentially removes most of the microbes that produce Vitamin B12 and the soil that contains that vitamin and other minerals necessary for optimal human health.

Another thing that humans generally refuse to do is consume feces, which is a relatively common practice among the other surviving great apes like chimpanzees, bonobos, orangutans and gorillas. Since the bacteria in the lower gut of great apes produce Vitamin B12, this may be one important way that those non-human relatives of ours get the B12 they need.

How much B12 humans need for good health depends on their age and current B12 status, but it is generally a miniscule amount. Humans are also very limited in the amount of B12 they can absorb orally by the amount of intrinsic factor they produce in their digestive system, so B12 injections are sometimes used for deficiency cases. For an adult human, a daily amount of 2.4 micrograms of B12 is considered absorbable and adequate to avoid deficiency symptoms like pernicious anemia.

While this tiny amount is so small as to be invisible to the human eye, B12 still has several important functions in the human body. Furthermore, since B12 is stored in the human liver and is recycled very efficiently, most adults can go for around 5 years without showing deficiency symptoms, although children do not have that safety buffer and may show deficiency symptoms more rapidly if their dietary intake of B12 is insufficient.

For those reasons, a B12 supplement or a daily multivitamin that includes at least 2.4 micrograms of B12 is strongly suggested for children and for anyone else intending to follow the Pliocene Diet on a long term basis. Since B12 is water soluble and an excess can be readily excreted in the urine, overdoses are rare.

Another major change in the human palate is the general rejection of insects as a desirable food source among modern humans, even if bugs only comprise a few percent of the diet of other great apes. This change tends to reduce the amount of omega 3 fatty acids in the human diet that include the key brain nutrients eicosapentaenoic acid (EPA) and docosahexaenoic acid (DHA) compared to what our ancestors may have eaten in the Pliocene Epoch.

Fortunately, most modern humans can convert the omega-3 fatty acid alpha-linolenic acid (ALA) contained in flax oil and walnuts to EPA and DHA as an alternative to consuming insects. Those who find they have a poor ALA conversion rate can instead source the EPA and DHA they need from algal oil that is obtained from marine algae. Taking an algal oil supplement can therefore be beneficial if any temporary reduction in memory or brain functioning is observed while on the Pliocene Diet as a result of EPA/DHA deficiency.

Another way in which modern humans tend to differ from their Pliocene ancestors is that they tend to get far less sunlight exposure. Since humans can manufacture the essential Vitamin D3 they need when sunlight hits their skin, a lack of sunlight exposure can result in a Vitamin D3 deficiency that can reduce the health of their bones and teeth unless it is supplemented. Fungi, such as mushrooms, do provide a decent dietary source of Vitamin D2, but it is just not as effective as D3 in humans. Accordingly, those who do not get at least 15 minutes of sun exposure between the hours of 10 am and 2pm each day should consider taking a D3 supplement obtainable from lichen. Keep in mind that D3 is a fat soluble vitamin and an excess cannot be readily excreted, so an overdose should not be taken.

An optional supplement some Pliocene Dieters may wish to consider is Vitamin B7 or biotin that contributes to strengthening hair and nails. If you will be eating more plant derived food and less food from animals on the Pliocene Diet, then you may notice that your hair and nails get weaker and break off more readily.

If you think about it, this would actually be a better adaptation for our ancestors in the Pliocene era since they did not have scissors to cut their excess hair or clippers to trim their long nails with, so those auxiliary body parts just broke off naturally to avoid potentially problematic overgrowth. Nevertheless, humans in the modern era might be used to their strong nails and thick hair. In that case, adding a regular B7 supplement can help keep nails and hair strong for cosmetic reasons if that is desired while on the Pliocene Diet.

Furthermore, although raw plant foods are packed with essential micronutrients and immune system-boosting vitamin C, it generally makes sense to take a daily multivitamin to cover all of the essential micronutrients and minerals necessary for optimal human health just in case. Drinking mineral water and consuming mineral salts like Himalayan pink salt can be helpful in getting all the minerals you need while on the Pliocene Diet.

Pliocene Diet Shopping Tips

Since all foods suitable for the Pliocene Diet are uncooked and unprocessed, make sure you are not buying anything packaged in a can that will have been heated during the canning process. Also take care to avoid food that has been combined in processing with unsuitable foods, such as all animal products, so be sure to read labels carefully.

Probably the best way to shop for foods suitable for the Pliocene Diet is to browse among the simple, fresh plant-derived items typically found in the Produce Section and bulk bins of your local grocery store. In general, avoid all canned foods, frozen vegetables that are usually blanched before freezing, any processed foods with more than one ingredient on the label, and foods that have had preservatives added to them. Also avoid packaged foods like plant based milks that are easy and less expensive to make at home.

Fatty whole foods like coconuts, olives and avocados are preferable to extracted oils, although flax and algal oils can be used as Omega 3 fatty acid supplements suitable for Pliocene Dieters. Also, since eating less is generally preferable when it comes to oils, you can choose to buy them only in small quantities to reduce your access to these indulgent high-calorie foods. Ideally, you will want to make sure their bottles have words like "extra virgin", "cold-pressed" and "first cold press" on them to make sure they have not been heated.

Also, certain specialty items are most easily purchased online if you do not have access to a health food store that carries them. They include truly raw cashews (most are steamed), raw almonds (most are pasteurized) and cold-pressed algal oil.

Pliocene Diet Flow Chart

Figure #1 shown on the following page contains a flow chart you can memorize and use while shopping to make decisions about a particular food item and whether or not it would be suitable for a Pliocene Dieter. You can memorize it, take a copy with you when you are shopping and/or post it on your refrigerator for easy reference.

Pliocene Diet Flowchart

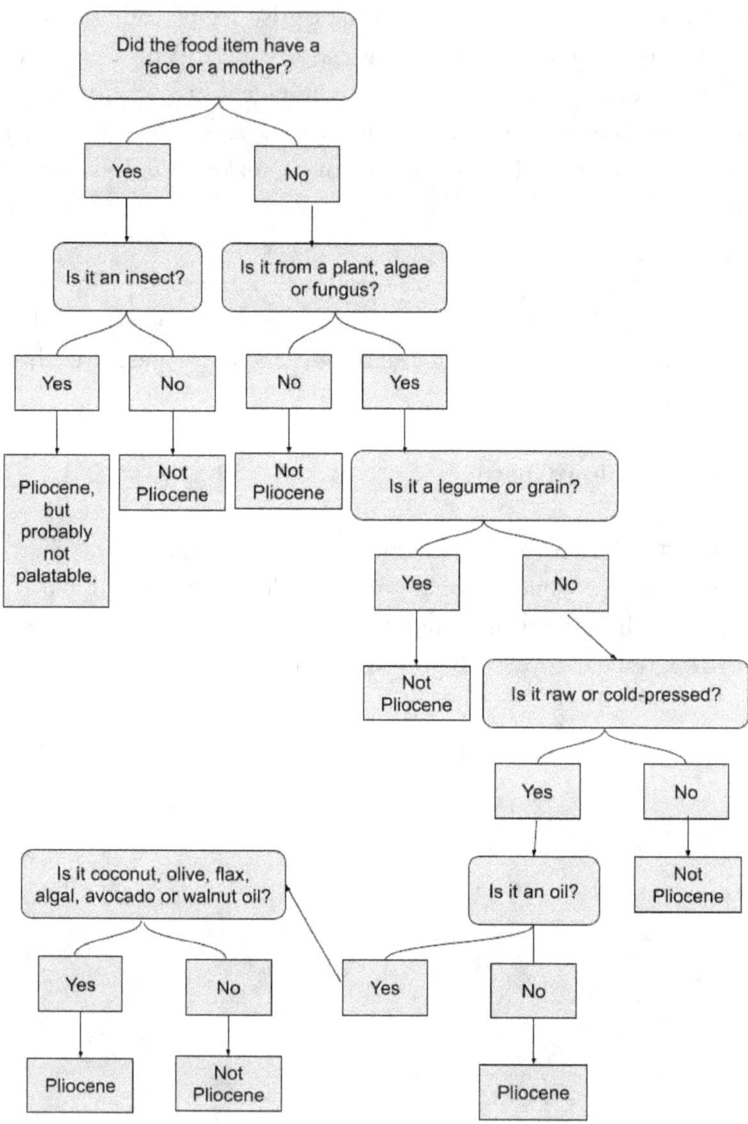

Figure #1: Flowchart showing how to decide if a particular unprocessed food item is suitable for the Pliocene Diet. Keep in mind that all processed or cooked foods are unsuitable.

Combining Food for Peak Nutrition on the Pliocene Diet

Among those with sensitive digestive systems who wish to strictly follow the Pliocene Diet, understanding the science of effective food combining is generally helpful. This section explains the key principles and strategies underpinning best food combining practices, offering insights into the cultivation of optimal nutrition and digestive equilibrium.

In the Pliocene Diet, the total absence of animal products, processed foods, oils, and legumes and grains directs the dieter's attention instead to a delicious palette of raw fruits, vegetables nuts, and seeds. The synergy among these diverse food groups and how to combine them properly becomes paramount, since it influences nutrient absorption and overall physiological balance.

Commencing this culinary exploration with a burst of freshness, the consumption of juicy fruits takes center stage. Best enjoyed on an empty stomach, these tasty fruits experience especially rapid digestion, which generally minimizes digestive effort. The deliberate sequencing of placing them first in a meal prevents the fermentation of sugars when combined with slower-digesting foods, thereby laying the foundation for a more harmonious and complete digestive process. Melons are generally also best eaten alone.

Next up for consideration are the leafy greens which have an especially vital role in the Pliocene Diet. Happily, they offer a profusion of micronutrients and enzymes to help you maintain optimal health. Ideally incorporated mid-meal or as a prelude to heartier components, the alkaline nature of leafy greens complements the acidity of fruits, contributing to a more balanced internal pH ideal for human health.

Finally, nuts and seeds are repositories of healthy fats and proteins, so they also feature prominently in this dietary regimen, although in moderate amounts kept to around 10% of the diet. However, their optimal digestion demands that they be kept separate from fruits to avert potential fermentation issues. Thorough chewing also becomes imperative, since it not only crushes the food but also facilitates the release of enzymes needed for its efficient breakdown.

A thoughtful approach to raw food pairing also amplifies the nutritional bounty contained in elements of the Pliocene Diet. For example, combining vitamin C-rich fruits with iron and calcium-laden leafy greens, for instance, augments the absorption of those essential minerals. This intentional and healthful combination enhances the bioavailability of essential nutrients, thereby fostering a more comprehensive nourishing experience.

Fluid dynamics also play a significant role in food combining. Hydrating food elements like cucumber, celery, and the water-rich fruits contribute to maintaining optimal fluid balance in your body. Strategic liquid consumption also ensures adequate hydration without diluting your digestive enzymes, thereby supporting the seamless function of the human digestive process.

Respecting digestive intervals should also be kept in mind as a cornerstone practice if you have a sensitive digestion. Creating temporal spaces between meals, particularly those with varying digestion rates, helps facilitate the effective assimilation of nutrients. This deliberate pacing honors the body's inherent rhythm when processing foods, thereby promoting greater digestive efficiency.

Remember to keep your interest in food active by allowing your culinary creativity to flourish. Explore different textures, flavors, and nutritional profiles of fruits, vegetables, nuts and seeds to allow for a more diverse and satisfying array of raw plant-based meals while on the Pliocene Diet. It is through this exploration that you can discover the rich array of possibilities within the defined parameters of this most natural ancestral dietary lifestyle.

The image on the following page shows how Pliocene Diet food combining works for optimal digestion. You will note that it puts melons off to the side since they are to be eaten alone, while leafy greens can be eaten along with all of the other plant food groups, including sweet, subacid and acid fruits; starchy and non-starchy vegetables; and fatty fruits, nuts and seeds.

Also take note that the overlaps of the circles show food groups that can be eaten together, while a lack of an overlap shows two food groups that should ideally not be consumed at the same time. For example, the fatty fruit group does not overlap with the sweet fruit group, so you might avoid eating foods from those groups together.

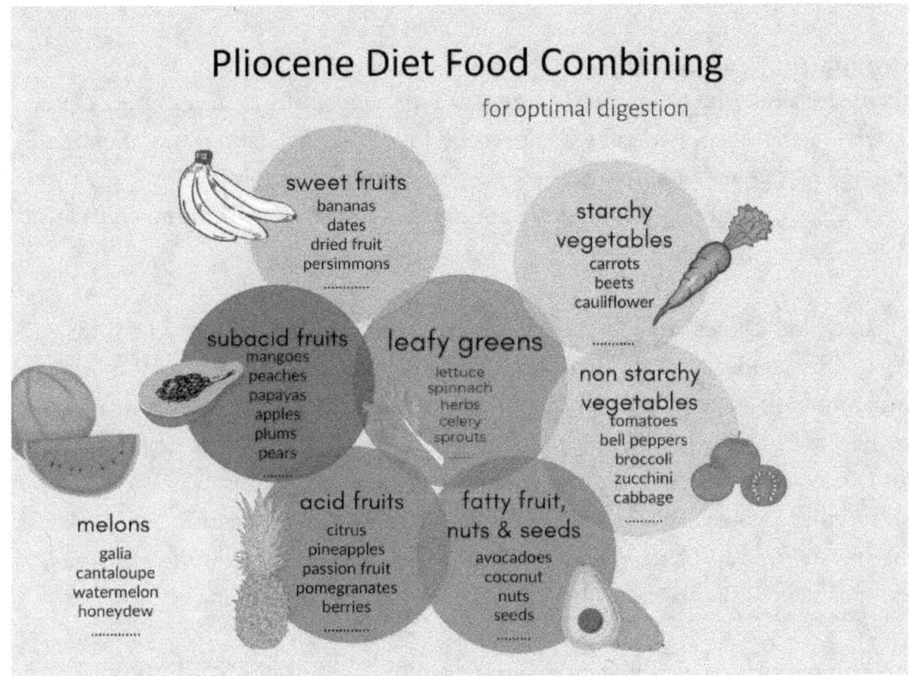

Figure #2: Diagram of optimal food group combining on the Pliocene Diet.

In conclusion, keep in mind that those with sensitive digestions may need to gain a more nuanced understanding of food combining principles to fully thrive on and enjoy the Pliocene Diet. Mastery of these principles will empower you to start your path towards sustained health on the Pliocene Diet with greater confidence as you enjoy the intricate dance of flavors, textures, and nutrients that characterize this ancestral dietary lifestyle.

Fighting Inflammation by Watching your Omega 3 to 6 Ratio

Three types of unsaturated fatty acids are contained in foods and are known as Omega 3, 6 and 9 fatty acids. Omega-3 fatty acids are polyunsaturated because they have many double bonds that cause a weakness in their molecular chain, and their first double bond is the third molecular bond. Omega-6 fatty acids are also polyunsaturated, and they have their first double bond at the sixth molecular bond. Omega-9 fatty acids are either monounsaturated or polyunsaturated, and they have their first double bond at the ninth molecular bond.

Only the Omega 3 and 6 fatty acids are essential for humans to get from their diet since they can make Omega 9 fatty acids. Monounsaturated Omega 9 fatty acids like oleic acid are present in olives, avocados and their cold-pressed oils that are suitable for Pliocene Dieters. Research shows they may have health benefits[13] that include strengthening the human immune system's response to pathogens.

Pliocene Dieters mainly need to focus on managing the ratio of Omega 3 to 6 fatty acids in their diet because Omega 3 fatty acids tend to reduce inflammation in the human body, while Omega 6 fatty acids tend to increase it. Research shows[14] that the ratio of these two essential fatty acids in foods and the quality of your diet in general can determine how much you suffer from the ravages of excessive inflammation. Inflammation can play a significant role in heart disease, arthritis, depression, Alzheimer's disease and even cancer. Inflammation also contributes to premature aging.

Humans and their Pliocene Epoch hominid ancestors probably evolved on a low inflammation diet with approximately an Omega 3:6 fatty acid ratio of 1. Modern research[15] also suggests you want to maintain at least a 1:4 or 0.25 Omega 3:6 ratio for maintaining good health by keeping inflammation in check. In standard Western diets, that ratio is more like 1:15 to 1:17, so it is far from what would be considered healthy. That notable excess of Omega 6 fatty acids generally leads to widespread inflammation in the human body that poses various serious health risks and causes early aging.

To keep your Omega 3 to 6 fatty acid ratio within the healthy range while on the Pliocene Diet, you need to know what that ratio is within the available nuts and seeds and then adjust your intake of those items accordingly. The

---

[13] https://www.ncbi.nlm.nih.gov/pubmed/23278117

[14] https://www.health.harvard.edu/staying-healthy/what-is-inflammation-and-why-is-it-dangerous

[15] https://www.health.harvard.edu/staying-healthy/what-is-inflammation-and-why-is-it-dangerous

two tables on the following page contain the Omega 6:3 ratio of various nuts and the Omega 3:6 fatty acid ratio of various seeds. Note that the ratios are inverted between the two groups. Also, peanuts have an especially poor Omega 6:3 ratio, and since they are legumes anyway, they are generally not suitable for Pliocene Dieters.

Walnuts, flax, chia and hemp seeds are among the best dietary sources of Omega 3 fatty acids, while algal oil and flax oil are very useful supplements suitable for Pliocene Dieters that you can take to balance the consumption of nuts or seeds with a poor Omega 3:6 ratio, such as almonds, for example. You may also note that seeds typically have better Omega 3:6 ratios than nuts, but certain seeds are definitely better than others in this regard, especially flax, chia and hemp seeds.

Nuts:

	Omega 3 Fats	Omega 6 Fats	Omega 6:3 Ratio
Walnuts	8.49	35.7	4.20
Macadamia nuts	0.196	1.3	6.63
Pecans	0.986	20.6	20.89
Cashews	0.161	7.66	47.58
Pistachios	0.289	14.1	48.79
Hazelnuts	0.087	7.83	90.00
Pine nuts	0.164	33.2	202.44
Almonds	0.052	14.5	278.85
Brazil Nuts	0.036	23.9	663.89
Peanuts	0.01	17.2	1720.00

Seeds:

Seed	Fat in 100g	Omega 3 (g)	Omega 6 (g)	Omega 3:6 ratio
Flax	42.2	22.81	5.91	3.8596
Chia	30.8	17.55	5.79	3.0311
Hemp	50	8.33	30	0.2777
Sesame	49.7	0.38	21.37	0.0178
Pumpkin	19.4	0.077	8.6	0.0090
Sunflower	51.5	0.074	23.05	0.0032

CHAPTER 7: PLIOCENE DIET FOOD PREPARATION

Throughout human history, people have developed a variety of methods and tools for preparing and preserving food. A few examples of ancient food preparation methods and tools that Pliocene Dieters can still use today include grinding with stone tools, fermenting, pickling, processing, dehydrating, soaking and sprouting.

These are just some of the many ancient food preparation methods and tools that have been used throughout history. Many of these methods and tools are still in use today, and they have been adapted and improved upon over time.

Since the Pliocene Diet is based on the most natural ancestral human diet, it uses various methods of food production that date back to ancient times. Each food preparation method, its relevance to Pliocene Dieters and the tools required to implement it will be described further in the following sections of this chapter.

Grinding:

Requires a grinding tool or machine.

One of the earliest methods of food preparation involved using stone tools to grind, chop, and pound food. This included using a grinding stone and base or a mortar and pestle to grind nuts and seeds into flour, or using a stone knife to chop vegetables. Grinding using stone tools or mortar and pestle is a food preparation method that has been used by humans for thousands of years and generally involves crushing and breaking down food items into smaller particles. This method of food preparation is commonly used for preparing spices, herbs, seeds, and flours, as well as for making pastes, dips, and sauces.

While coffee grinders, flour grinders, and food processors are the modern appliances of choice for this purpose, if you want to use more traditional methods, you could instead use stone tools made from volcanic rock. An example is the molcajete that is used in preparing salsa, guacamole and other sauces and dips used in traditional Mexican cuisine. This grinding device can be obtained in Mexico, from Mexican stores elsewhere and online.

Furthermore, a mortar and pestle are used to make curry pastes in Thai cuisine, for example. To use a mortar and pestle, the food item is placed in the mortar, which is a bowl-shaped container made from stone. The pestle, which is a rounded stone or wooden tool, is then used to crush and grind the food item by pressing and grinding it against the sides and bottom of the mortar. The repeated motion of grinding breaks the food item down into smaller pieces until it reaches the desired consistency.

Grinding using stone tools or mortar and pestle has several advantages. Firstly, it allows for precise control over the size and texture of the ground food, which can influence the flavor and texture of the final dish. Secondly, it can help release the natural oils and flavors of the food item, which can enhance the taste and aroma, especially for aromatic spices. Lastly, it is a simple and effective method that requires no electricity or other modern equipment, making it a very natural, sustainable and accessible food preparation method suitable for Pliocene dieters.

Soaking:

Requires a waterproof bowl and drinking water.

Soaking nuts and seeds in water is an ancient food preparation method that involves placing raw nuts and seeds in a waterproof container and covering them with water. The water is typically room temperature or slightly warmer, and drinking water can be used for this process. The nuts and seeds are then left to soak for a certain period of time, usually between 4-12 hours, depending on the type of nut or seed.

During the soaking process, the water penetrates the outer layer of the nuts and seeds, which activates enzymes and breaks down phytic acid. Phytic acid is a compound found in nuts and seeds that can inhibit the body's ability to absorb nutrients such as iron, calcium, and zinc. Soaking the nuts and seeds can help to reduce the amount of phytic acid, thereby making the nutrients more bioavailable.

Soaking nuts and seeds also makes them easier to digest, as it softens them and reduces the amount of work the digestive system has to do to break them down. Additionally, some people find that soaking nuts and seeds can improve their texture and flavor.

After soaking, the nuts and seeds are typically rinsed and drained before using them in recipes, such as adding them to smoothies, making nut milk, or using them as a topping for salads or in raw granola recipes. Soaking is also generally the precursor step to sprouting.

It is important to note that some nuts and seeds, such as cashews, flax, chia and pumpkin seeds, can become slimy when soaked for too long. It is also important to discard the soaking water, since it may contain anti-nutrients and toxins that have been released from the nuts and seeds during the soaking process.

Sprouting:

Requires jar with mesh top for small batches or mesh bowl with cover for larger batches.

Sprouting seeds is a food preparation method that involves soaking and then draining seeds and then exposing them to air and moisture until they begin to sprout. This method can be done using jars or mesh bowls.

To sprout seeds using jars, the seeds are first rinsed and then soaked in a jar filled with water for several hours, depending on the type of seed. The water is then drained and the jar is tipped upside down and propped at an angle to allow excess water to drain out. The jar is then covered with a piece of cloth or mesh to keep the seeds from drying out and to allow air to circulate. This process is repeated several times a day until the seeds have sprouted to the desired length.

To sprout seeds using a mesh bowl, the seeds are rinsed and then placed in a bowl with mesh lining. The bowl is then placed on a tray or dish to allow excess water to drain out. The seeds are then covered with a piece of cloth or mesh to keep them from drying out and to allow air to circulate. The seeds are then rinsed several times a day until they have sprouted to the desired length.

Sprouting seeds is a simple and cost-effective way to increase the nutritional value of seeds. Sprouts are a good source of vitamins, minerals, and enzymes, and they are easily digestible. Sprouting can also increase the bioavailability of certain nutrients and make them easier to absorb.

Sprouts can be added to salads, nori rolls and other raw dishes, or eaten as a nutritious snack on their own. However, it is important to handle sprouts safely, as they can be a source of foodborne illness if they are not handled properly.

It is generally recommended to rinse sprouts thoroughly before eating them and to store them in the refrigerator. Additionally, pregnant women, the elderly and people with weakened immune systems should avoid eating raw sprouts to reduce the risk of contracting a foodborne illness.

Processing:

Requires chewing or machines like food processors and blenders.

Food processing is a method of food preparation that involves breaking down food into smaller pieces or changing its texture using various techniques and tools. Some common food processing methods include chewing, using a food processor or using a blender.

Chewing is a natural food processing method that involves using the teeth and jaws to break down food into smaller pieces. Chewing is important because it helps to mix food with saliva, which contains enzymes that start the process of digestion. Chewing also makes food easier to swallow and digest.

Using a food processor or blender is a more mechanical food processing method that involves using an electric or manual device to chop, blend or puree food. Food processors and blenders have various blades and attachments that can be used to chop vegetables, grind nuts and seeds, blend smoothies or puree soups. These devices can be particularly useful for making the sauces, dips and purees used in some Pliocene Diet recipes.

Food processing using a blender or food processor can also make food easier to eat and digest, since it breaks down the food into smaller pieces or changes its texture. This can be especially beneficial for people with tooth problems and those who have difficulty chewing or swallowing.

Additionally, food processing can make it easier to incorporate a variety of raw fruits, vegetables, nuts and seeds into the Pliocene diet, since they can be blended into smoothies or pureed into tasty sauces and dips. However, it is important to note that some food processing methods, such as juicing fruits and vegetables, can remove some of the fiber and other nutrients found in the whole food. Also, any form of processing that results in heating the food above 117 degrees F is to be avoided to retain optimal nutrition from raw plant foods.

Finally, remember to avoid store-bought processed food that has added sugars or other undesirable ingredients for Pliocene Dieters that may be included by food processing companies. It is typically best to only buy whole or minimally processed plant foods whenever possible and to do any desired food processing at home. This generally means shopping only for whole foods in the produce sections and bulk bins of a grocery store and preparing your own meals at home.

Dehydrating:

Requires sun drying or a hot air dehydrator with a temperature setting.

Dehydrating is a method of food preparation that involves removing moisture from food to help preserve it for longer periods of time and change its texture. This method can be done using the sun or a hot air dehydrator with a temperature setting.

Sun drying is a traditional method of dehydrating food that involves laying food out in the sun to dry. This method works best in hot, dry climates with low humidity. Fruits, vegetables and herbs can all be sun-dried. However, sun-drying can be a slow process, taking several days to complete, and can be affected by weather conditions.

A hot air dehydrator is a modern device that uses a fan and heat source to dry food quickly and efficiently. These devices typically have temperature settings that can be adjusted to achieve the desired level of dehydration. Fruits, vegetables, herbs, seeds and nuts can all be dehydrated in a dehydrator.

Dehydrating food is a raw food preparation method because it involves using low temperatures to preserve the natural enzymes and nutrients found in food. This can make dehydrated foods a great option for people who are following a raw food diet.

Dehydrated foods can be stored for long periods of time and can be used in a variety of ways. Dehydrated fruits can be eaten as snacks, added to cereals or granolas, or used in baking. Dehydrated vegetables can be rehydrated and used in soups, stews, and other dishes. Dehydrated herbs can be used as seasoning or to make herbal teas.

It is important to note that some dehydrated foods may be high in sugar or sodium, especially if they are commercially produced. Additionally, it is important to follow proper food safety guidelines when dehydrating food to prevent the growth of bacteria and other harmful pathogens.

Fermenting:

Requires a fermenting container and starter culture.

Fermenting food is an ancient method of raw food preservation that has been used for thousands of years. It involves allowing beneficial bacteria, fungi and yeasts to break down sugars and other nutrients in food, creating lactic acid, alcohol and other compounds that help preserve the food.

Fermenting is a popular method for preserving raw fruits and vegetables, as well as for creating yogurts out of nut milks and fermented teas like kombucha. Other fermented foods include sauerkraut and kimchi.

The process of fermenting can improve the nutritional quality of foods, as it can increase the bioavailability of vitamins, minerals, and other nutrients in the food. Fermented foods are also known to promote gut health, as they can contain beneficial bacteria that can help to improve digestion and boost the immune system.

To ferment food, the raw ingredients are typically chopped or shredded and mixed with a starter culture or naturally occurring microorganisms, such as those found on the surface of fruits and vegetables. The mixture is then left to sit at room temperature for several days to several weeks, depending on the food being fermented and the desired level of fermentation.

During the fermentation process, the microorganisms convert the sugars in the food into lactic acid and other compounds, which create an acidic environment that helps to preserve the food. The acid also gives fermented foods their tangy flavor.

Some examples of fermented raw foods include:

- **Sauerkraut:** a fermented cabbage dish that is high in vitamin C and fiber.
- **Kimchi:** a Korean fermented vegetable dish that is usually made with cabbage, radishes, and spices.
- **Kombucha:** a fermented tea that is made with a symbiotic culture of bacteria and yeast (SCOBY).
- **Nut and Seed Cheezes:** Raw, fermented nut and seed products such as almond milk yogurt and sunflower seed cheeze.

It is important to note that not all fermented foods are considered raw, as some are pasteurized or cooked prior to the fermentation process. When preparing fermented raw foods at home, it is important to follow proper food safety guidelines to avoid contamination with harmful bacteria.

Pickling:

Requires pickling container and salt or vinegar.

Pickling is another ancient method of food preservation that involves soaking food in a solution of vinegar or brine. This helps to preserve the food by creating an acidic environment that inhibits the growth of bacteria.

Pickling is another raw food preparation method that has been used for thousands of years to help preserve food. It does this by using acid or vinegar to create an environment that inhibits the growth of harmful bacteria.

To pickle raw vegetables or fruits, the first step is to prepare the ingredients by washing and cutting them into desired sizes. The next step is to create a pickling solution, which usually includes vinegar, salt, sugar, and various spices and herbs for flavoring. In many cases, commercial picklers boil the pickling solution before pouring over the prepared vegetables or fruits, which are then packed into clean jars or containers. This step needs to be avoided if possible by Pliocene Dieters since it heats the food.

The equipment required for pickling includes the pickling jars or containers which should be made of non-reactive materials, such as glass or ceramic, since reactive materials like metal can react with the acid in the pickling solution and affect the flavor and safety of the pickles. Additionally, the jars or containers should have an airtight seal to prevent air from entering and contaminating the pickles.

Once the jars or containers are filled with the pickling solution and vegetables or fruits, they should be allowed to cool to room temperature before being stored in a cool, dark place. Over time, the acid in the pickling solution will penetrate the vegetables or fruits and create an environment that inhibits the growth of harmful bacteria. This allows the pickles to be stored for several months or even longer.

Some examples of raw foods that are commonly pickled include cucumbers, beets, carrots, onions and garlic. Pickled vegetables can be enjoyed as a snack, added to salads or sandwiches, or used as a condiment to add flavor to dishes.

In addition to the pickling jars or containers, the equipment required for pickling may include a large pot for making the pickling solution, a ladle for pouring the pickling solution into the jars or containers, and a canning funnel to prevent spills. Other optional equipment may include a mandoline or sharp knife for slicing the vegetables, and a kitchen scale to measure ingredients accurately.

CHAPTER 8: THE PLIOCENE DIET TRANSITION

Transitioning to the Pliocene Diet can be a significant lifestyle change. This diet involves consuming uncooked, unprocessed, pre-agricultural and ideally organic plant-based foods, such as fruits, vegetables, nuts and seeds.

If you are considering transitioning to the Pliocene Diet, then there are several things you should keep in mind to ensure a smooth and healthy transition. Each of these transition guidelines will be covered in the following sections.

Educate Yourself

Before making any significant dietary changes, it is generally important to educate yourself on the benefits and challenges of the new diet you are embarking upon, and starting the Pliocene Diet is no exception to that rule.

You can start out on your Pliocene Diet journey by reading any books, websites and articles you can find on ancestral plant-based diets. You have already taken an initial step in that direction by reading this introductory book on the topic!

Another educational path could involve attend workshops and lectures by experts on the Pliocene Diet and plant-based ancestral diets in general. You can even seek advice from experienced Pliocene Dieters, as well as from raw vegans who have a similar uncooked and unprocessed plant-based diet.

Getting Started with Your Transition

Transitioning to a new diet, even an ancestral one like the Pliocene Diet, can be challenging, especially if you are used to eating cooked foods and animal products. It is important to set realistic goals for yourself, such as gradually increasing the amount of raw foods in your diet over a few weeks or months.

Starting with small changes will make it easier for you to adjust to the new diet gradually and sustainably. The following sections include some useful tips on how to set realistic goals when transitioning to a raw plant-based diet.

Assess Your Current Diet

Before setting any goals, it is essential to assess your current diet and identify areas that need improvement. Take a look at your current eating habits, the types of foods you consume, and your daily calorie intake. This will help you set specific goals that are tailored to your individual needs.

Start Small

Transitioning to a raw vegan diet can be a significant change, so it is important to start small and gradually increase the amount of raw foods in your diet. For example, you could start by incorporating one raw meal a day, such as a raw salad or a green smoothie, and gradually increase the number of raw meals over time.

Consider Your Lifestyle

When setting goals, it is essential to consider your lifestyle and schedule. If you have a busy work schedule or travel frequently, it may be challenging to follow a strict Pliocene Diet.

Instead, you can consider setting realistic goals that are achievable, such as increasing the amount of raw plant foods you consume on weekends or when you have more time to prepare meals.

You can also take a pack lunch with you when you know you will not be able to get suitable foods at work. Deep salad greens, fresh fruit and dehydrated crackers tend to keep for quite some time in an airtight plastic container. Avocadoes, nuts and seeds are also excellent travel foods that are very satisfying due to their fat content.

When it comes to eating out at restaurants, you can usually call ahead to see if the culinary staff can accommodate your dietary needs either right off the menu or with a special order. If not, you can probably choose another restaurant to patronize instead that can serve the food you prefer.

Stay Flexible

It is important to be flexible when setting goals for your new dietary lifestyle. While the Pliocene Diet is very healthy, it is probably not realistic to expect yourself to follow it strictly all the time.

Unless you are changing your diet for ethical reasons because you care deeply about farmed animals and their welfare, you may want to allow yourself some flexibility to indulge in animal products occasionally. The same general principle applies to occasionally indulging in cooked plant foods if you cannot get raw plant foods.

The need for some dietary flexibility is especially understandable if you are dining out with friends, family, clients or colleagues and do not wish to make a fuss by asking for special food.

Still, always keep in mind that you can usually just choose to fast temporarily until raw plant foods are again available, much like your Pliocene ancestors would have done. While you cannot survive a week without water, you can live for months without food.

Set SMART Goals

When setting goals for your new Pliocene Diet lifestyle, it is important to make them SMART. This acronym stands for: Specific, Measurable, Attainable, Relevant and Time-bound. Setting SMART goals means you should try to set goals that are:

(1) *Specific:* Make goals clear and specific so that you know exactly what you should be doing,

(2) *Measurable:* Make goals measurable so that you know when you are attaining your goals or failing to do so,

(3) *Attainable:* Goals should be achievable so that you will not be disappointed due to certain failure,

(4) *Relevant:* Goals need to be relevant to your lifestyle and health goals so that you are not sidetracked from achieving what is truly important to you, and

(5) *Time-Bound:* Your goals should have a certain specified timeline that you intend to meet them within.

Celebrate Your Successes

As you achieve your goals, it is important to celebrate your successes. Celebrating your achievements will help you stay motivated and make it easier to maintain your new diet in the long run. You can throw yourself a success party or just have some friends or a special someone over for a Pliocene dinner to celebrate.

In summary, setting realistic goals when transitioning to the Pliocene Diet requires assessing your current diet, starting small, considering your lifestyle, staying flexible, setting SMART goals and celebrating your successes. By setting achievable goals and making gradual changes, you can successfully transition to you true ancestral diet and enjoy the many health benefits the Pliocene Diet provides.

Plan Your Meals

Planning your meals in advance will help you ensure that you are getting all the nutrients you need from your raw vegan diet. Before you go shopping, resolve to make a list of your favorite raw fruits, vegetables, nuts and seeds, and plan your meals around them.

Strictly avoid buying anything that does not conform to Pliocene Diet guidelines when you go shopping. Remember that it is generally easier to stop your cravings at the store that than try to ignore a non-conforming food item when you are looking at it in your cupboard or refrigerator.

You can also experiment with new recipes and raw plant food preparation techniques to keep your Pliocene meals interesting and nutritious.

Start Slowly

Most dieticians do not recommend switching to a raw plant-based diet overnight if you are not largely eating that way already. While some people are still willing to transition sharply, they often have to go through the resulting gut flora die-off reaction that can make them feel a bit ill for a few days.

This reaction happens because you do not just feed yourself when you eat food, but you also feed a plethora of bacteria that live in your digestive tract. When you no longer feed those microbes the animal products and cooked food they expect, they tend to die off and release toxins in the process that your body needs to expel. We tend to interpret that detoxifying process as an illness, although we are in fact getting rid of microbes and their products that are often not beneficial to us and can contribute to disease.

Instead of risking having a detox reaction, you can start transitioning to the Pliocene Diet gradually by adding more raw plant foods to your current diet each day while cutting out more and more animal products and cooked plant foods as you do so. For example, you can start your day with a green smoothie or a raw fruit salad for breakfast. You can then have a raw salad with nuts and seeds for lunch. You can then eat some components of your previous diet for dinner.

If you do decide to use this gradual transition method, you should plan on slowly reducing the amount of cooked foods and animal products you consume over a specific amount of time until you are fully transitioned to the raw Pliocene Diet.

Stay Hydrated

Fortunately, the Pliocene Diet is typically high in water-rich foods, such as fruits and green leafy vegetables, which can help keep you hydrated during your transition.

However, it is still important to attend to your hydration needs by drinking plenty of water throughout the day to prevent dehydration. You can also drink herbal teas, fresh juices or coconut water to help stay hydrated.

Also, if your digestion is moving too quickly on the new diet, which can also lead to dehydration, then you can add foods like ginger, shredded coconut or coconut paste, and drinks like green tea that tend to slow your digestion down.

Supplement When Necessary

While the Pliocene Diet provides so many health benefits, it can also be challenging to get all the nutrients you need from raw plant foods you are not used to eating and so do not know the nutritional value of. Fortunately, virtually anyone who is eating enough calories each day will not have to worry about getting enough of the macronutrients that consist of fat, protein and carbohydrates.

Micronutrients, such as vitamins, minerals and essential fatty acids, are another matter, however. Even those eating conventional diets are often deficient in several of these important nutrients that help assure good health. At the very least, you should consider supplementing your Pliocene diet with vitamin B12 and omega-3 fatty acids from plant based sources like walnuts, flax or hemp seeds, and algal oil supplements, to help ensure that you are getting all the essential nutrients. You can also get tested on a periodic basis to make sure you have no important vitamin deficiencies.

Furthermore, those concerned about having unnaturally stronger hair and nails may want to supplement with biotin since the Pliocene Diet typically has more modest amounts. Finally, while your body does naturally synthesize vitamin D from exposure to direct sunlight or a special lamp, you should plan on getting a daily dose of at least 15-20 minutes between the hours of 10 am and 2pm or consider supplementing with that important vitamin instead.

Listen to Your Body

As with any dietary change, it is important to listen to your body and make adjustments as necessary. The vast majority of transition issues tend to be minor and resolve quickly once your body gets used to the new diet and your gut flora composition returns to a more natural state.

However, if you experience any notable negative side effects from the transitioning process — such as fatigue, a severe detox reaction that can feel a bit like the flu, and/or chronic digestive issues like constipation or diarrhea — please seriously consider researching the issue so that you can adjust your diet according to the best advice you can find or promptly consult with a healthcare professional to get those problems sorted out.

In summary, transitioning to the Pliocene Diet will very likely have great health benefits to you, as well as reducing any harm done to animals and the environment by your diet. Still, committing to consuming any raw vegan diet in the modern era of fast, cooked and processed "frankenfood" requires planning, patience, willpower and a persistent openness to experiment with the fresh foods and raw recipes that conform to your new diet.

By setting realistic goals, gradually increasing the amount of raw foods in your diet, and listening to your body, you can successfully and easily transition to the Pliocene Diet and lifestyle to start enjoying the many health benefits the most natural diet for your physiology readily provides.

PLIOCENE DIET MEAL PLANS AND RECIPES

CHAPTER 9: PLIOCENE DIET MEAL PLANS

You have probably already learned the general guidelines for following the Pliocene Diet by now just from reading the previous chapters of this book. Still, to get you started quickly on following this healthful ancestral diet so you can reap the many benefits of eating the best and most natural diet for your species, this chapter provides several examples of simple and delicious conforming meal plans.

You can use these eight sample meal plans as a general guide when transitioning to the Pliocene Diet, but do feel free to improvise based on your own tastes, caloric and nutritional needs, and food preferences.

Meal Plan 1:

Breakfast: Green smoothie made with kale, banana, peach and almond milk.
Morning Snack: Apple slices with raw almond butter.
Lunch: Large salad with mixed greens, cherry tomatoes, cucumber, avocado and a lemon-tahini dressing.
Afternoon Snack: Raw pumpkin seeds with sea salt.
Dinner: Zucchini noodles with tomato sauce made from blended sun dried tomatoes, walnuts, garlic and basil.

Meal Plan 2:

Breakfast: Chia seeds soaked overnight with almond milk topped with fresh berries and sliced raw almonds.
Morning Snack: Fresh fruit salad with mixed berries, mango and papaya.
Lunch: Collard green wrap filled with nut and seed paste, avocado, alfalfa

sprouts, red peppers and cucumber.

Afternoon Snack: Energy balls made with dates, raw nuts and seeds.

Dinner: Sushi made with cauliflower rice, avocado, cucumber and bell pepper wrapped in raw nori seaweed.

Meal Plan 3:

Breakfast: Parfait made with layers of young coconut creme, fresh berries and raw granola made from nuts, seeds and dried fruit.

Morning Snack: Fruit smoothie made with bananas, mango and coconut milk.

Lunch: Zucchini noodles with pesto made from basil, pine nuts, garlic and coconut crème.

Afternoon Snack: Pepper, cucumber, celery and squash sticks with guacamole.

Dinner: Pizza made with a dehydrated cauliflower and flax crust topped with a sundried tomato sauce, marinated onions and mushrooms, crushed raw spinach and chopped basil.

Meal Plan 4:

Breakfast: Acai bowl topped with fresh fruit, coconut flakes and chia seeds.

Morning Snack: Sushi made with avocado, cucumber and celery sticks on chopped cauliflower rice wrapped in raw nori seaweed.

Lunch: Taco salad made with a romaine lettuce base topped with sundried tomato chopped with walnut, avocado and a creamy young coconut and lemon dressing

Afternoon Snack: Kale chips dusted with sea salt.

Dinner: Pad Thai made with zucchini noodles, shredded cabbage, slivered peppers, chopped scallions, garlic, cilantro, soaked sunflower seeds, and a spicy nut sauce made with raw almond butter, nama shoyu sauce, lime juice and ginger.

Meal Plan 5:

Breakfast: Chia seed pudding made with almond milk, topped with fresh berries and sliced almonds

Morning Snack: Red grapes with a cantaloupe melon.

Lunch: Caesar salad made with romaine lettuce, cherry tomatoes and a creamy coconut dressing.

Afternoon Snack: Celery sticks with sunflower seed cheese.

Dinner: Lasagna made with layers of zucchini noodles, coconut ricotta cheeze, crushed spinach, and tomato sauce made from blended sun dried tomatoes, garlic and fresh basil.

Meal Plan 6:

Breakfast: Smoothie bowl made with blended acai, mixed berries, and almond milk, topped with fresh fruit and coconut flakes

Morning Snack: Energy balls made with dried cherries, coconut, nuts and seeds.

Lunch: Sushi rolls made with cauliflower rice, avocado, cucumber and bell pepper wrapped in raw nori seaweed.

Afternoon Snack: Raw almond butter and banana slices on flax crackers.

Dinner: Spaghetti made with zucchini noodles topped with raw tomato and chopped walnut marinara sauce.

Meal Plan 7:

Breakfast: Raw vegan granola made from chopped nuts, seeds and dried fruit, served with young coconut crème and fresh berries.

Morning Snack: Raw celery, pepper and cucumber sticks with guacamole.

Lunch: Raw vegan wrap made with collard greens, mushroom nut paste, avocado, red peppers and cucumber.

Afternoon Snack: Raw fruit smoothie made with bananas, strawberries and coconut milk.

Dinner: Raw vegan tacos made with chopped walnut and sun dried tomato meat, avocado, tomato, and a coconut and lemon sour crème sauce, served on romaine lettuce leaves.

Meal Plan 8:

Breakfast: Green smoothie made with spinach, mango, apple and almond milk.

Morning Snack: Raw California rolls made with avocado on chopped cauliflower wrapped in raw nori seaweed.

Lunch: Raw Greek salad made with mixed greens, cherry tomatoes, cucumber, purple onion, sunflower seed cheeze balls, and a creamy tahini dressing

Afternoon Snack: Soaked raw almonds with sea salt.

Dinner: Raw vegan pad Thai made with zucchini noodles and a spicy sauce made with raw almond butter, lime juice and ginger.

As these sample meal plans show, following the Pliocene Diet can be varied, delicious and nutritious experience! These meal plans are just examples of what you can eat on this raw plant food diet, and feel free to experiment with different ingredients to keep your meals interesting and satisfying. You can also customize the sample meal plans to fit your personal taste preferences and dietary needs.

Keep in mind that by incorporating a variety of raw fruits, greens, nuts and seeds into your diet in sufficient amounts to meet your personal caloric needs, you can ensure that you are getting all the essential nutrients your body needs for excellent health.

In case you sense a lack of a particular nutrient and/or start to have strong food cravings, you can always check that your customized Pliocene Diet meal plans and portions are adequate for your individual nutritional needs by entering them into a nutritional website like Cronometer.com.

CHAPTER 10: PLIOCENE DIET RECIPES

You may have noticed from the sample meal plans presented in the previous chapter that recipes for most of the food eaten by people enjoying the Pliocene Diet are quite self-explanatory. This is largely due to the fact that this natural and healthy ancestral diet mainly focuses on raw fruits and greens with some nuts and seeds added for their fat and protein content.

Still, some of our delicious Pliocene Diet recipes are a bit more complex, so a sampling of those recipes have been provided below for your convenience, along with some additional tasty recipes for your dining pleasure. Happily, these recipes are flavorful, nutritious and quite easy to make. Enjoy!

Nori Rolls:

Ingredients:

1 Nori sheet
1/2 avocado
1/2 cucumber, thinly sliced
1/2 red pepper, thinly sliced
1/2 celery stick, thinly sliced
1/4 red onion, thinly sliced
1/2 cup alfalfa sprouts
1 cup finely chopped cauliflower
Sesame seeds

Instructions:

(1) Place the Nori sheet shiny side down on a sushi mat or a piece of plastic wrap.
(2) Put a 1 inch wide band of chopped cauliflower sideways across the nori sheet.

(3) Arrange the vegetables and sprouts on top of the cauliflower band.
(4) Sprinkle sesame seeds on top of the vegetables.
(5) Roll the nori sheet tightly, using the sushi mat or plastic wrap to help.
(6) Wet the top edge of the nori with a little water and press to seal.
(7) Use a sharp knife to cut the roll into bite-size pieces.
(8) Serve with ginger and a savory dipping sauce.

Caesar Salad:

Ingredients:

1 head of romaine lettuce, chopped
1/4 cup coconut crème
2 tbsp. lemon juice
1 Medjool date
1 garlic clove, minced
1/4 cup water
Salt and pepper to taste

Instructions:

(1) Rinse and chop the romaine lettuce and set aside.
(2) In a blender or food processor, combine the coconut crème, lemon juice, date, garlic and water. Blend until smooth and creamy.
(3) Pour the dressing over the chopped lettuce and toss to coat evenly.
(4) Season with salt and pepper to taste.
(5) Serve immediately.

Pad Thai:

Ingredients:

2 medium zucchinis, spiralized into noodles
1/2 cup sliced red cabbage
1/4 cup slivered pepper
1/4 cup chopped scallions
1/4 cup chopped cilantro
1/4 cup soaked sunflower seeds
Juice of 1 lime
2 tbsp. raw almond butter
2 tbsp. savory sauce

1 Medjool date
1 tbsp. grated ginger
1 garlic clove, minced
3 tbsp. water
Salt and pepper to taste

Instructions:

(1) In a large bowl, combine the spiralized zucchini and sliced red cabbage.
(2) In a separate bowl, whisk together the lime juice, almond butter, savory sauce, date, grated ginger, minced garlic, water, salt and pepper.
(3) Pour the sauce over the vegetable mixture and toss to coat evenly.
(4) Garnish with chopped cilantro, scallions and sunflower seeds.
(5) Serve chilled.

Zucchini Pasta with Tomato Sauce:

Ingredients:

2 medium zucchinis, spiralized into noodles
2 large tomatoes, chopped
1/4 cup sun-dried tomatoes, soaked in water for 10 minutes
1/4 cup soaked walnuts
1 garlic clove, minced
1/4 cup fresh basil leaves
1 tbsp. avocado
1/4 tsp sea salt
1/4 tsp black pepper

Instructions:

(1) Spiralize the zucchinis into noodles and set aside.
(2) In a food processor, finely chop the tomatoes, soaked sun-dried tomatoes, walnuts, minced garlic, basil leaves, olive oil, sea salt, and black pepper. Blend until smooth.
(3) Put the tomato sauce onto the zucchini pasta and toss to coat evenly.
(4) Serve immediately.

Green Smoothie Bowl:

Ingredients:

1 banana
1 cup mango chunks
1/2 avocado
1/2 cup coconut water
2 cups baby spinach
1/4 cup fresh mint leaves
1 tbsp. chia seeds
1 tbsp. hemp seeds
Fresh fruit, raw granola or nuts for topping

Instructions:

(1) In a blender, combine the banana, mango chunks, avocado, coconut water, baby spinach and fresh mint leaves. Blend until smooth.
(2) Pour the smoothie into a bowl and top with chia seeds, hemp seeds and your choice of fresh fruit, raw granola or nuts.
(3) Serve immediately.

Almond Date Energy Balls:

Ingredients:

1 cup raw almonds
1 cup dates, pitted
1/4 cup unsweetened shredded coconut
1 tsp ground cinnamon
1/4 tsp ground nutmeg
1/4 tsp sea salt

Instructions:

(1) Combine all ingredients in a food processor. Pulse until the mixture is crumbly but can be pressed together.
(2) Use your hands to shape the mixture into bite-size balls.
(3) Serve immediately or place the energy balls in the refrigerator to store.

Carrot Noodles with Avocado Pesto

Ingredients:

5 large carrots, spiralized
1 ripe avocado
1/2 cup fresh basil leaves
1/4 cup pine nuts
2 cloves garlic
1 tbsp. lemon juice
Salt and pepper to taste

Instructions:

(1) Place the spiralized carrot noodles in a large bowl.
(2) In a blender or food processor, blend avocado, basil, pine nuts, garlic, lemon juice, salt and pepper until smooth.
(3) Pour the pesto over the carrot noodles and toss to coat.

Creamy Broccoli, Raisin and Sunflower Seed Salad:

Ingredients:

2 cups broccoli florets
1/2 red onion, thinly sliced
1/4 cup raisins
1/4 cup soaked sunflower seeds
1/4 cup lemon juice
1 date
1 tbsp. water
1 tsp ground mustard seeds
1/4 cup young coconut crème
Sea salt and black pepper, to taste

Instructions:

(1) In a large bowl, combine the broccoli florets, red onion, raisins and sunflower seeds.
(2) In a small bowl, whisk together the lemon juice, date, water, ground mustard seeds and coconut crème until well combined.
(3) Pour the dressing over the broccoli mixture and toss to coat evenly.
(4) Season with sea salt and black pepper to taste.
(5) Chill the broccoli salad in the refrigerator for at least 30 minutes before serving.

Raw Carob Mousse:

Ingredients:

1 ripe avocado
1/4 cup raw carob powder
1/2 cup water
3 Medjool dates
1 tbsp. soaked almonds
1 tsp ground dried vanilla bean
Pinch of sea salt

Instructions:

(1) In a food processor or blender, combine the ripe avocado, raw carob powder, dates, water, almonds, vanilla bean and sea salt.
(2) Blend until the mixture is smooth and creamy.
(3) Spoon the chocolate mousse into serving dishes.
(4) Chill the chocolate mousse in the refrigerator for at least 30 minutes before serving for a thicker consistency.

Strawberry Cheezecake:

Ingredients:

For the crust:

1 cup soaked raw almonds
1/2 cup pitted Medjool dates
1/4 cup shredded coconut
1/4 tsp sea salt

For the filling:

2 cups raw macadamia nuts, soaked in water for at least 4 hours
1/2 cup young coconut crème
1/3 cup water
5 Medjool dates
1/2 cup fresh lemon juice
1 tsp ground vanilla bean
1/2 cup fresh strawberries, chopped

Instructions:

(1) In a food processor, pulse the raw almonds, pitted Medjool dates,

shredded coconut and sea salt until the mixture forms a sticky dough.

(2) Press the dough into the bottom of a 9-inch spring form pan.

(3) In a blender, combine the soaked raw macadamia nuts, coconut crème, water, dates, fresh lemon juice and vanilla. Blend until the mixture is smooth and creamy.

(4) Pour half of the filling mixture over the crust.

(5) Add the chopped strawberries to the remaining filling mixture in the blender and blend until smooth.

(6) Pour the strawberry filling over the first layer of filling.

(7) Use a spatula to smooth the top of the cheesecake.

(8) Chill the raw vegan strawberry cheesecake in the refrigerator for at least 4 hours, or until set.

(9) Slice and serve the cheesecake cold.

Zucchini Strips with Creamy Avocado Alfredo Sauce:

Ingredients:

2 medium zucchinis, sliced into thin strips with a potato peeler
1 ripe avocado
1/4 cup fresh basil leaves
1 clove garlic, minced
2 tbsp. lemon juice
2 tbsp. coconut crème
Sea salt and black pepper, to taste

Instructions:

(1) In a large bowl, toss the zucchini strips with sea salt and let sit for 10 minutes to soften.

(2) In a food processor or blender, combine the ripe avocado, fresh basil leaves, minced garlic, lemon juice, coconut crème, sea salt and black pepper.

(3) Blend until the mixture is smooth and creamy.

(4) Pour the creamy avocado Alfredo sauce over the zucchini strips and toss to coat evenly.

(5) Serve immediately.

Raw Butternut Squash Soup:

Ingredients:

2 cups of peeled and chopped butternut squash
1 small red onion, roughly chopped
2 cloves garlic, minced
1 tbsp. fresh ginger, grated
2 cups coconut milk
1 tbsp. coconut crème
Sea salt and black pepper, to taste

Instructions:

(1) In a high-speed blender, blend the chopped squash, red onion, minced garlic, grated ginger, coconut milk and crème, sea salt, and black pepper until the mixture is smooth and creamy. If you blend it enough, it will warm up.

(2) Pour the butternut squash soup into serving bowls.

(3) Serve immediately.

Cherry Coconut Energy Bites:

Ingredients:

1 cup pitted Medjool dates
1 cup unsweetened shredded coconut
1 cup dried cherries
1 cup soaked nuts and/or seeds
1/4 cup water
1/4 tsp sea salt

Instructions:

(1) In a food processor, pulse the pitted Medjool dates, unsweetened shredded coconut, dried cherries, soaks nuts and seeds, and sea salt until the mixture is well combined and forms a sticky dough.
(2) Using your hands, roll the dough into small balls.
(3) Place the energy bites on a baking sheet lined with parchment paper.
(4) Serve immediately or place in the refrigerator to store.

Zucchini Noodles with Pesto:

Ingredients:
2 zucchinis, spiralized into noodles

1 cup fresh basil leaves
1/4 cup raw pine nuts
1/4 cup coconut crème
1 clove garlic
1/4 tsp sea salt
Juice of 1 lemon

Instructions:

(1) In a food processor or blender, combine the fresh basil leaves, raw pine nuts, coconut crème, garlic, sea salt, and lemon juice.
(2) Blend until the mixture forms a smooth pesto sauce.
(3) Toss the zucchini noodles with the pesto sauce until evenly coated.
(4) Garnish with additional pine nuts and fresh basil leaves, if desired.
(5) Serve immediately.

Fruit Salad with Citrus Dressing:

Ingredients:

2 cups mixed tart fresh fruit, such as strawberries, blueberries, raspberries and sliced kiwi.
Juice of 1 orange
Juice of 1 lemon
1 tbsp. date syrup
1 tbsp. coconut crème

Instructions:

(1) In a large bowl, combine the mixed fresh fruit.
(2) In a small bowl, whisk together the orange juice, lemon juice, date syrup and coconut crème until well combined.
(3) Pour the citrus dressing over the fruit and toss to coat evenly.
(4) Serve immediately.

Grated Apple and Walnut Salad:

Ingredients:
2 cups grated apple
1/4 cup raisins
1/4 cup chopped walnuts
1 tbsp. lemon juice
1 tbsp. coconut crème

2 tsp date syrup
Sea salt and black pepper, to taste

Instructions:

(1) In a large bowl, combine the grated apple, raisins, and chopped walnuts.
(2) In a small bowl, whisk together the lemon juice, coconut crème, date syrup, sea salt and black pepper until well combined.
(3) Pour the dressing over the apple, raisin and walnut mixture and toss to coat evenly.
(4) Serve immediately or store in the refrigerator.

Coconut Chia Pudding:

Ingredients:

1 cup coconut milk
1/4 cup chia seeds
2 tbsp. date syrup
1 tsp ground vanilla bean
Pinch of sea salt

Instructions:

(1) In a medium bowl, whisk together the coconut milk, chia seeds, date syrup, vanilla bean and salt so that the chia seeds are evenly distributed.
(2) Cover and refrigerate overnight.
(3) Stir once more in the morning to evenly combine the seeds.
(4) Taste and add more date syrup if you'd prefer it sweeter.
(5) Put a serving into your bowl, and then add your favorite toppings.

Cucumber Avocado Gazpacho

Ingredients:

2 cucumbers
1 avocado
1/2 cup of water
1/4 cup of lemon juice
1 garlic clove

1/4 cup of fresh cilantro

Instructions:

(1) In a blender, combine cucumbers, avocado, water, lemon juice, garlic and cilantro.
(2) Blend until smooth
(3) Serve chilled and garnish with diced cucumber and cilantro leaves

Very Berry Sorbet:

Ingredients:

2 cups mixed berries (such as strawberries, raspberries and blueberries)
1/2 cup unsweetened almond milk
1/4 cup date syrup
1 tsp ground vanilla bean

Instructions:

(1) In a blender, combine the mixed berries, unsweetened almond milk, date syrup and ground vanilla bean.
(2) Blend until the mixture is smooth and creamy.
(3) Pour the berry mixture into a container and freeze for at least 2 hours.
(4) Use a spoon or ice cream scoop to serve the berry sorbet.

Beet and Carrot Salad

Ingredients:

2 large beets, peeled and grated
3 large carrots, peeled and grated
1/4 cup chopped fresh parsley
1/4 cup chopped fresh cilantro
1/4 cup chopped fresh mint
2 tbsp. coconut crème
1 tbsp. lemon juice
Sea salt and pepper to taste

Instructions:

(1) In a large bowl, combine grated beets, grated carrots, parsley,

cilantro and mint.

(2) In a separate bowl, whisk together olive oil, apple cider vinegar, salt and pepper.

(3) Pour the dressing over the beet and carrot mixture and toss to combine.

Carrot Ginger Soup:

Ingredients:

2 cups of chopped carrots
1 small red onion, roughly chopped
2 cloves garlic, minced
1 tbsp. fresh ginger, grated
2 cups coconut milk
1 tbsp. coconut crème
Sea salt and black pepper, to taste

Instructions:

(1) In a high-speed blender, blend the chopped carrots, red onion, minced garlic, grated ginger, coconut milk and crème, sea salt, and black pepper until the mixture is smooth and creamy. If you blend it enough, it will warm up.

(2) Pour the carrot ginger soup into serving bowls.

Serve immediately.

Creamy Cauliflower Rice:

Ingredients:

1 head cauliflower
1/2 cup chopped fresh parsley
1/4 cup chopped fresh mint
2 tbsp. coconut crème
2 tbsp. lemon juice
Sea salt and pepper to taste

Instructions:

(1) Cut the cauliflower into small pieces and place in a food processor.

(2) Pulse the cauliflower until it resembles rice.

(3) Transfer the cauliflower rice to a large bowl and add chopped parsley and mint.

(4) In a separate bowl, whisk together the coconut crème, lemon juice, salt and pepper.

(5) Pour the dressing over the cauliflower rice and toss to combine.

Veggie Rolls:

Ingredients:

1 large cucumber, peeled and cut into thin strips
1 large carrot, peeled and cut into thin strips
1 large red bell pepper, seeded and cut into thin strips
1 avocado, sliced
1/4 cup chopped fresh cilantro
1/4 cup chopped fresh mint
6 dehydrated coconut wrappers

Instructions:

(1) Place the dehydrated coconut wrapper on a flat surface. Wet as needed to make it pliable.

(2) Layer cucumber, carrot, red bell pepper, avocado, cilantro and mint in the center of the wrapper.

(3) Fold the sides of the wrapper over the filling, and then roll it up tightly.

(4) Repeat with remaining ingredients.

Broccoli, Cranberry and Walnut Salad:

Ingredients:

1 head broccoli, chopped into small florets
1/4 cup chopped red onion
1/4 cup chopped dried cranberries
1/4 cup chopped walnuts
2 tbsp. coconut crème
2 tbsp. lemon juice
Salt and pepper to taste

Instructions:

(1) In a large bowl, combine broccoli florets, red onion, dried cranberries and walnuts.
(2) In a separate bowl, whisk together olive oil, lemon juice, salt and pepper.
(3) Pour the dressing over the broccoli salad and toss to combine.

Carrot Cake Bites:

Ingredients:

1 cup raw macadamia nuts
1 cup shredded carrots
1/2 cup dates, pitted
1/4 cup unsweetened shredded coconut
1 tsp ground cinnamon
1/4 tsp ground nutmeg
1/4 tsp ground ginger
1/4 tsp sea salt
1 tbsp. coconut crème

Instructions:

(1) In a food processor, combine the raw nuts, shredded carrots, pitted dates, shredded coconut, cinnamon, nutmeg, ginger, sea salt and coconut crème.
(2) Pulse until the mixture is crumbly but can be pressed together.
(3) Use your hands to shape the mixture into bite-size balls.
(4) Serve immediately or store in the refrigerator.

Raw Tacos:

Ingredients:

1 head romaine lettuce
1 avocado, diced
1 small red onion, diced
1 small tomato, diced
1 small red bell pepper, diced
Juice of 1 lime
Salt and pepper to taste

Instructions:

(1) Wash and dry the romaine lettuce leaves, and use them as the taco shells.
(2) In a large bowl, combine the diced avocado, red onion, tomato, and red bell pepper.
(3) Add lime juice, salt, and pepper to taste, and mix well.
(4) Spoon the vegetable mixture into the lettuce taco shells.
(5) Serve immediately.

Cabbage, Carrot and Beet Salad:

Ingredients:

1 cup shredded red cabbage
1 cup shredded carrots
1 cup shredded beets
1/4 cup chopped fresh parsley
1/4 cup chopped fresh mint
1/4 cup lemon juice
1/4 cup coconut crème
1/4 tsp sea salt
1/4 tsp black pepper

Instructions:

(1) In a large bowl, toss together cabbage, carrots, beets, parsley, and mint.
(2) In a separate bowl, whisk together the lemon juice, coconut crème, sea salt and black pepper.
(3) Pour the dressing over the salad and toss to combine.
(4) Serve chilled.

Cucumber and Tomato Salad:

Ingredients:

2 medium cucumbers, sliced
2 medium tomatoes, chopped
1/4 cup chopped red onion
1/4 cup chopped fresh dill
2 tbsp. lemon juice
2 tbsp. coconut crème
Sea salt and pepper to taste

Instructions:

(1) In a large bowl, toss together cucumbers, tomatoes, red onion and dill.
(2) In a separate bowl, whisk together lemon juice, coconut crème, sea salt and black pepper.
(3) Pour the dressing over the salad and toss to combine.
(4) Serve chilled.

Red Beet and Carrot Slaw:

Ingredients:

2 medium beets, grated
2 medium carrots, grated
1 cup red cabbage, grated
1/4 cup lemon juice
1 tbsp. poppy seeds
1/4 cup coconut crème
1/4 tsp sea salt
1/4 tsp black pepper

Instructions:

(1) In a large bowl, toss together beets, carrots, cabbage and poppy seeds.
(2) In a separate bowl, whisk together lemon juice, coconut crème, salt, and black pepper.
(3) Pour the dressing over the slaw and toss to combine.
(4) Serve chilled.

Tomato Basil Soup

Ingredients:

4-5 large tomatoes
1/2 cup of soaked macadamia nuts
1 garlic clove
1 tbsp. of lemon juice
1/4 cup of fresh basil
1/4 cup of water

Instructions:

(1) In a blender, combine tomatoes, nuts, garlic, lemon juice, basil and water.
(2) Blend until smooth.
(3) Serve chilled or at room temperature.

Carrot Cucumber Soup:

Ingredients:

6 medium carrots, peeled and roughly chopped
1 medium cucumber, peeled and roughly chopped
1 cup fresh orange juice
1 tbsp. grated ginger
Sea salt and pepper to taste

Instructions:

(1) In a blender, blend the carrots, cucumber, orange juice, ginger, salt, and pepper until smooth.
(2) Warm in blender or serve chilled.

Tangy Cucumber Onion Salad:

Ingredients:

2 medium cucumbers, peeled and thinly sliced
1 medium red onion, thinly sliced
2 tbsp. lemon juice
1 tbsp. date syrup
Sea salt and pepper to taste

Instructions:
(1) In a large bowl, mix the cucumbers and red onion.
(2) In a separate bowl, whisk together the lemon juice, date syrup, salt and pepper.
(3) Pour the dressing over the cucumber mixture and toss to coat.
(4) Serve chilled.

Sweet Potato Noodle Salad:

Ingredients:

2 medium sweet potatoes, peeled and spiralized
1 large red bell pepper, thinly sliced
1 medium red onion, thinly sliced
2 tbsp. raw tahini
2 tbsp. freshly squeezed lemon juice
1 tbsp. date syrup
Sea salt and pepper to taste

Instructions:

(1) In a large bowl, mix the sweet potato noodles, red bell pepper and red onion. In a separate bowl, whisk together the tahini, lemon juice, date syrup, salt and pepper.
(2) Pour the dressing over the sweet potato mixture and toss to coat.
(3) Serve chilled.

Garlic Cauliflower Mashed Potatoes:

Ingredients:

1 medium head of cauliflower, roughly chopped
2 tbsp. of freshly squeezed lemon juice
3 tbsp. coconut crème
3 cloves garlic
Sea salt and pepper to taste

Instructions:

(1) In a food processor, process all ingredients until it resembles mashed potatoes.
(2) Serve immediately.

Raw Burrito Wrap

Ingredients:

4 large collard green leaves
2 ripe avocados, mashed
1/2 red pepper, diced
1/2 onion, diced
1/2 tomato, diced
1/4 cup of cilantro, chopped

Juice of 1 lime
Salt and pepper to taste
1/2 cup walnuts and sun dried tomatoes

Instructions:

(1) Remove the tough stems from the collard green leaves and place them on a plate.
(2) In a bowl, combine the mashed avocado, red pepper, onion, tomato, cilantro, lime juice, salt and pepper to create a filling.
(3) Process the walnuts and sundried tomatoes into a coarse paste.
(4) Place a line of the walnut and sundried tomato paste on each collard green leaf, spoon the filling on top of that line, and wrap it up like a burrito.
(5) Serve immediately.

Rainbow Salad:

Ingredients:

1 cup shredded red cabbage,
1 cup grated carrots,
½ cup sliced bell pepper,
½ cup chopped kale
2 tbsp. Macadamia nuts
1 tbsp. lemon juice
1 clove garlic
Sea salt and pepper to taste

Instructions:

(1) Toss cabbage, carrots, pepper and kale ingredients together in a salad bowl.
(2) Blend nuts, lemon juice, garlic, salt and pepper, then pour on salad and massage into other ingredients.
(3) Serve immediately.

ABOUT THE AUTHOR

After obtaining her physical science degrees, Alice Dee studied nutritional healing and herbology for decades. In addition to growing a thriving food forest, she also founded a pioneering raw plant-based restaurant in Northern California. Alice is the author of various other books related to plant-based diets, as well as the organizer of related online forums. She is available for speaking and consulting on the Pliocene Diet and other topics related to plant-based nutrition.

For more information, please visit her websites at

www.PlioceneDiet.com

www.NutritionalHealer.com

www.RawFromTheGarden.com

www.TheFoodForestGuide.com

www.PeakPerformanceDiet.com

For fully raw plant-based recipes suitable for Pliocene Dieters that you can make grocery store-bought whole foods and produce from your garden, you can buy Alice's restaurant-tested Raw Vegan Recipes book here:

www.RawVeganRecipesBook.com

For additional support as a Pliocene Dieter, you can join Alice's large and active Raw Vegan Recipes Facebook Group here:

www.facebook.com/groups/rawveganrecipes1/

www.ingramcontent.com/pod-product-compliance
Lightning Source LLC
Chambersburg PA
CBHW050738260726
48661CB00001B/299